Overcoming Common Problems

Dementia

Everything your doctor doesn't have time to tell you

DR MATT PICCAVER

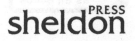

sheldon PRESS

First published in Great Britain by Sheldon Press in 2020
An imprint of John Murray Press
A division of Hodder & Stoughton Ltd,
An Hachette UK company

This paperback edition published in 2020

1

A CIP catalogue record for this title is available from the British Library

Paperback ISBN 9781847094827
eBook ISBN 9781847094810

Typeset by Cenveo® Publisher Services.

Printed and bound in Great Britain by Clays Ltd, Elcograf S.p.A.

John Murray Press policy is to use papers that are natural, renewable and
recyclable products and made from wood grown in sustainable forests. The
logging and manufacturing processes are expected to conform to the
environmental regulations of the country of origin.

John Murray Press
Carmelite House
50 Victoria Embankment
London EC4Y 0DZ

www.sheldonpress.co.uk

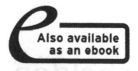

Also available
as an ebook

Contents

Acknowledgements

To my family and friends and those I love and have loved, thank you for your support during the writing of this book. To my children Ted and Lewis, who keep me grounded, occupied, and repeatedly bruised. They are a couple of wonderful, energetic, and amusing kids and I love them all dearly.

This book is dedicated to all those diagnosed with dementia. Yours is a difficult path, and I hope this book goes some way to helping guide you along it. To all carers, both professional and informal. Looking after a person with dementia isn't easy. While their reality diverges from yours, it's difficult to retain a sense of perspective, or remember why you do that job. This book is for you. To the army of family carers, who spend hours and hours in a day with their loved ones, helping fill the gaps that form in life as dementia gets worse. This book is for you. I only ever have about ten minutes with a patient at any one time, you have weeks, months and even years.

To the platoons of health care professionals, nurses, doctors, physiotherapists, occupational therapists, speech and language therapists, podiatrists (have I missed anyone out?) who are involved in the care of people with dementia. This book is for you.

Thanks to my publisher for putting up with countless delays, particularly as the day job has been so utterly hectic throughout the writing of this book. Finally, thanks to you for taking the time to read it, particularly as you probably have better things to do and are probably really rather busy.

Introduction

As a GP I've met countless people over the course of my career. All human life eventually finds its way to my door. All strata of society, at some point, need the help of a doctor. We are none of us immune from the ravages of disease, time or disability.

I'll try not to sound too bleak. As a GP I've got ten short minutes to assess, diagnose and treat a condition. It doesn't really matter what that condition might be. A serious diagnosis might hinge on a single sentence. The 'door handle diagnosis', a diagnosis made as the person I'm seeing mentions something on the way out. Ten minutes to meet and greet. Ten minutes to allay fears or confirm suspicions. Ten minutes to provide reassurance, or give life-changing news.

What can you do in ten minutes? It takes that long for my kids to get out the door to go to school (they do it five days a week, so why does it come as a surprise that they need to wear shoes or need their school bag?). I've had baristas take longer than that to make a coffee. Fair enough, it might have been a fairly elaborate frappuccino, plus breakfast toastie. Oh, and a granola pot. And probably a biscuit. You get the point. It isn't long enough to do anything meaningful for anyone.

This book is there to fill in the gaps. A diagnosis like Alzheimer's, or any form of dementia, takes much longer than ten minutes. The ramifications of such a diagnosis are life long. As a doctor there are lots of things I need to tell people in order to help them understand or come to terms with their diagnosis. Being diagnosed with an illness such as Alzheimer's is a scary proposition for many of us. It can radically alter the rest of our lives, and those of our loved ones. It can put a strain on relationships, and have physical, emotional, social and even financial consequences.

This book aims to help people understand their diagnosis, and help those around them learn how to approach the care of someone with dementia.

As a doctor, I've met countless people with dementia. My first experience was a long time before medical school. I lived on a 1970s housing estate in the East of England. Rows of houses, and for some reason each half of the road was named something different. The 'streets' were named after the bits of grass in between the houses, called 'walks', and the roads were merely rear access to the properties. I'm not sure why, but in the seventies it seemed popular to build housing estates that caused the inhabitants or visitors to become utterly confused. I'm surprised we ever received any post. For those of us living there, it seemed perfectly natural. Since I've been a GP, I've been repeatedly lost in estates like this. Roads nowhere near houses, en masse garage blocks obscuring views of the house or street, dark alleyways and blind bends. I have a terrible sense of direction, and I like to think I'm relatively free of diseases affecting my brain.

Given the labyrinthine nature of my childhood haunts, perhaps it was not surprising that, one day, my mother and I found an elderly lady outside the back of the house. Or perhaps it was the front. It's hard to tell. She looked rather disorientated. My mother asked her where she needed to be. Rather coincidentally, my mother had a letter for that very address that she needed to post, and we walked with the lady back to her home. Either that, or we walked her to a complete stranger's property and let her in. We never did find out what happened, but we assumed this to be the lady's house. In retrospect, I suspect this lady was suffering from dementia, and most likely Alzheimer's disease. Disorientation in usually familiar environments is one symptom that might point the way to a diagnosis of dementia. Either that or, like many visitors to our estate, she wasn't entirely certain where she was.

Alzheimer's, and in fact all types of dementia, make up a very common group of conditions. It's difficult not to find a person who doesn't know someone who has dementia, or who might be caring for a loved one with the disease. In this book we'll talk about what Alzheimer's disease is, and touch upon other forms of dementia. We will look at what we can do to try to prevent the condition developing. We will look at some of the signs and symptoms of Alzheimer's. Is there anything we might be able to spot before it takes hold? We will talk about the sorts of tests and investigations that might be needed, as well as any treatments that might help. We will look at medications, and non-drug treatments, as well as complementary therapies. We'll provide tips about how to live well with dementia, to make the most of life regardless of the diagnosis given. Finally, we will look at some of the current research and see what hopes we might have for future treatments.

A diagnosis of dementia can be a scary prospect for people and their families. This book aims to take some of the mystery away, shed a little light on the dark corners and, hopefully, provide a little reassurance along the way.

1

Your amazing brain

Alzheimer's disease is one of a group of conditions called neuro-degenerative diseases. Neuro referring to the brain, and degenerative is self-explanatory. There are a number of different neuro-degenerative diseases including Alzheimer's disease, Huntington's disease, Parkinson's disease and motor neurone disease.

These conditions affect people in different ways, but one of the things they have in common is they all cause bits of the nervous system, be it centrally in the brain or peripherally in the nerves, to no longer work correctly. If they don't work properly, neither do we, and this goes some way to explaining why we find what we do in people suffering from such diseases.

Alzheimer's is part of a family of conditions that cause dementia. There are a number of different types of dementia. Perhaps the one I see most is Alzheimer's, but we also have vascular dementia, dementia with Lewy bodies, frontotemporal dementia, alcohol-related dementia, Creutzfeldt-Jakob Disease (CJD), as well as mixed dementia types (e.g. vascular/Alzheimer's simultaneously). We also see dementia in Parkinson's disease, Niemann-Pick's disease (type C), HIV-related cognitive impairment and Progressive Supranuclear Palsy. Some of these conditions are more common than others. We'll briefly touch on these other conditions in a later chapter. The main subject of this book is dementia and how to live with such a diagnosis.

Before we go into the subject of what exactly dementia is, I'm going to tell you a little bit more about your brain.

Your brain is amazing. It's a grey and white, squidgy blanc-mange of amazingness. A kilogram and a bit of brilliance, and each and every one of us has one. A supercomputer capable of amazing calculations, recall and recognition. Able to process countless signals from the nerves that run to and from our brain to our bodies.

Everything is in our heads. The colour orange. The smell of freshly mown grass. The taste of lemons. Happiness and sadness, joy and sorrow, pain and pleasure are all processed by the brain. Our sense of self, our hopes and dreams, our beliefs and prejudices all happen in that collection of billions and billions of neurons. Every action, want, need and desire comes, in part, from the brain. When a person asks me if something is 'in their heads', my answer is, 'yes, along with everything else'. We are, in part, a walking, talking, life support machine for the contents of our craniums. Our species is incredible. Arguably one of the most adaptable species on the planet, able to tame nature, reach for the stars, and make a complete hash of more or less everything we attempt to do in the process. We are brilliantly terrible, and terribly brilliant in equal measure.

Every amazing discovery, every catastrophic war, every moment of joy and sorrow originates in the brain. Pretty mind blowing, isn't it?

Take a minute to sit and look around you. Think about the things your brain needs to be able to do. What do you see? Light enters your eye, hits your retina, and a signal conveyed by the optic pathway to your occipital lobe, and processed by the brain to form a visual image.

What can you hear? A ticking clock? Birds singing? In my house it's usually my kids.

Air pressure, causing our eardrums to vibrate, activating tiny bones called ossicles, which causes the hair cells of the cochlear to move about, a signal relayed by our auditory nerve where our brain processes this information and recognizes this sensation as sound.

Take a sniff? Odours are detected in our olfactory bulbs, with fibres poking down into the top of our noses through a paper thin piece of bone called the cribriform plate, which is then conveyed to our brains and interpreted as scent.

Think about a time when you were happy. It might have been the birth of a child, a graduation, a time spent doing something fun with the people you love. I can recall the birth of my children as if it were yesterday. When I think back to those times, I can conjure up the sights and sounds, and even those feelings of fear, worry and, ultimately, untapped joy as if it were happening now. These memories make me what I am today, and their value is immeasurable. All of this is happening thanks to my brain. We are the product of our deeds, both good and bad. We are the product of our experiences, our upbringing and our genes. Our brain is shaped by our experiences and our environment, to make us who we are today.

All our five senses have an ability to trigger memories, emotions and sensations. Multiple connections between different parts of our brains give meaning, memory and emotion to practically every interaction we have. We learn from each experience, we understand what lemons smell like, what happiness feels like, what happened a week last Tuesday. You get the point. Your brain makes you who you are. Alzheimer's, in fact I would argue all dementia and neuro-degenerative diseases, rob us of what makes us who we are. Perhaps that sounds a little melodramatic, perhaps a bit too much of a sweeping statement but, if our brains make us who we are, then perhaps it is entirely understandable that when bits of it work less well, who we are changes. Slowly, over time, becoming evident to those around us.

We all change throughout our lives. I like to think most people are fairly open minded. Perhaps just the ones I meet. Our sense of the world changes as we experience life. Attitudes and beliefs evolve over time as we experience more and more of what life brings us. I'm pretty convinced that none of us share the same thoughts about life, the universe and everything that we had as children, teenagers or young adults. There is nothing permanent about us, or our experiences, and our ideas will flux. Who we are changes with our experience of life.

Before we delve into Alzheimer's, I'm going to tell you a little more about this amazing brain of yours. First some facts and figures. Your experience of your little patch of the universe is processed by an organ weighing about 1.4 kg. That's almost one bag and a half of sugar. There are thought to be 100 billion neurons in the human brain. A neuron is the name given to an individual nerve cell and the cells are, in essence, the building blocks of life, especially ours. Nerve cells are rather special things. They have a cell body, surrounded by dendrites, like little roots connecting with other cells. Leading from this body is the axon. Imagine it as like a wire conducting electrical signals down to synapses. Synapses are at the end of cells, and contain chemicals called neurotransmitters. Like a microscopic relay race, they pass the signal on to the next cell to carry out whatever task called upon them. Scaled up, these cells work together to allow us to think, feel, walk and talk, laugh and skip and jump and sing (should the fancy take you). Like all parts of the human body, they are truly amazing. I'm probably labouring the point now.

There are other cells in the brain too. Aside from neurons, there are cells known as glia. There are three types of glia, and they are: astroglia (astrocytes), oligoglia (oligodendrocytes) and, finally, microglia. I can recall at some point during my days at school being told that the glia didn't have a function, or that their function was largely unknown. However, with time comes scientific progress, and we now have some idea of what glia might do. Part of their role is involved in the immune system of the brain, and they kick into activity in the context of inflammation in the brain (the body's way of dealing with something it doesn't like), and neuro-degenerative diseases, of which Alzheimer's is just one. Glial cells are involved in the repair of damage, and given that for years these cells have been regarded as devoid of function, they are now subject to much study. We will discover more about what these cells do in the fullness of time (but not in the pages of this book, I hasten to add).

All of these cells work together to form the human brain; arguably one of the most sophisticated examples of evolution on the planet. The brain consists of several sections or lobes. There are lots of ways of referring to bits of the brain but, for the sake of brevity and because it has been so long since I studied neuro-anatomy, I'll keep it simple.

Basically, the outer part of the brain is called the cerebral cortex. It's the outer part, the folded bit that you see when you first take a peek inside someone's skull (we've all done that, right?).

The cortex is divided into lobes. The frontal lobe is at the . . . well, front. The occipital is at the back, the parietal on the sides and the temporal lobes at the temples. More deeply we have the limbic system, and towards the bottom of the brain we have the brain stem. This consists of lots of important parts that do things that we don't need to think too much about. They just happen, at least as far as we are concerned.

The frontal lobe is, in part, involved in control of movement, complex thoughts, how we get along in social environments, our inhibitions, impulses and behaviour. The parietal lobe is involved in perception, the occipital lobe is responsible, in part, for vision, and the temporal lobe is involved in hearing and smell.

Deeper to this is the limbic system, which consists of the hypothalamus, pituitary gland, the amygdala and the hippocampus. The hypothalamus and pituitary are important in the regulation of hormones which, you'll be pleased to know, we won't talk too much about in this book. The amygdala is important to survival, particularly when it comes to an awareness of fear, and the hippocampus is involved in the formation of memory. This is an important and yet fairly small part of the brain, at least where this book is concerned. In fact, I can't really think of any parts of the brain that aren't important. They're all there for a reason. Contrary to popular belief, we don't use a mere ten per cent of our brain. It's just that some people we meet in our daily lives might seem to.

This brilliant brain of yours is attached to a spinal cord, the main wiring loom that contains nerves leaving and entering the brain, allowing us to walk and talk, move and feel, run, hop, skip, and jump. Our thoughts are turned into actions, signals sent back down to our muscles to carry out our intentions. Unconscious processes permit us to breathe, digest our food, change our heart rate, or respond to danger or pain in a split second; out of our own control but there to keep us above ground for another day.

It is staggering to think just how much we can achieve with the human brain.

To paraphrase the late cosmologist Carl Sagan and his 'Pale Blue Dot' speech . . .

> Every feeling of love and hate, all of life's knowledge and work, the memories of people and places lost to us, every feeling of joy or suffering, every religious belief, act of heroism or cowardice, creation or destruction, invention or desire to

explore, every lesson learned, every misdeed committed, every work of art or symphony scored, every act of peace or war, every ideology, everything you've ever known or ever will know in part originated in a human brain.

If that doesn't blow your mind, nothing will.

2
What is Alzheimer's disease?

Alzheimer's is a member of a group of conditions referred to as neuro-degenerative. As we've mentioned previously, this means assorted parts of the brain degenerate, degrade, fall apart. They get smaller, or disappear, their neurons reduce in number, and if they aren't there, the brain doesn't work. Areas of our brain that once had function are no longer there to access, to carry out their role and make us who we are. It might be memories of people or places, or a mental set of instructions on how to carry out a certain task or how to navigate around our home town.

According to the World Health Organization, dementia is a group of conditions characterized by a reduction in memory, difficulty thinking, changes in behaviour and problems carrying out the activities of daily living. It is more common in older people but that doesn't necessarily make it a factor of normal ageing. There are an estimated 47 million people living with dementia worldwide, and around 10 million new cases are diagnosed every year. Alzheimer's makes up around 60 to 70 per cent of all cases.

Given that dementia causes so many problems with our ability to function, it is clear that this group of conditions are a major cause of disability and dependency across the globe. It causes physical problems, especially if we struggle to attend to our own care. It causes psychological problems in terms of depression, problems regulating behaviour or controlling our emotions. Dementia has a massive impact from a social perspective. It causes economic difficulties, and affects not just the patient but their families, carers, and society as a whole.

Dementia is a massive deal.

Dementia, and in particular Alzheimer's, is usually a long term, progressive condition. You might notice problems with memory, thinking, orientation in time and place, comprehension and understanding of language, difficulty with calculations and numbers, and judgement and decision making may become impaired. We may notice difficulties with emotional control, behaviour in social settings, or find a loss in motivation and drive. People with dementia can be left in a very vulnerable position indeed.

For many, the diagnosis of dementia can feel overwhelming, and I won't be lying in saying that some people I've met find it just that. Others will press on with life, adapting to the challenges that such a diagnosis brings, determined to get as much out of life as possible. The path we choose is, in part, dependent on many factors: how much support we have, our prior understanding of the condition, and perhaps how advanced it might be at the time of diagnosis. For some, the diagnosis of dementia brings with it a stigma, a feeling that they are no longer valuable, or can't engage with friends, family and colleagues in the ways they are used to. As we will discover over the course of this book, this doesn't have to be the case.

According to the Alzheimer's Society, there are around 850,000 people living in the UK with a diagnosis of a form of dementia (as of 2015), and the vast majority of those are aged over 65 years. Over one per cent of the UK population has dementia, and with the rate of population growth and ageing that we have experienced in the UK over the previous decades, it is estimated that as many as two million people will be living with dementia by the middle of the century. And around 115 million people worldwide. That's a lot of people potentially needing extra help and support. A lot of worried family members. A lot of family members spending their time caring for loved ones. A lot of stress, worry and anxiety.

Diagnosis rates of dementia have increased steadily over the past few decades. Around 60 per cent of cases are diagnosed as Alzheimer's, 17 per cent vascular dementia, 10 per cent mixed dementia, 4 per cent dementia with Lewy Bodies, 2 per cent frontotemporal, Parkinson's at around 2 per cent and 'other' at 3 per cent.

Now let me tell you a story. This is the tale of Alois Alzheimer, the scientist and doctor after whom Alzheimer's disease was named. In nineteenth century Germany Alois Alzheimer, in the course of his research, met a patient called Auguste Deter, a 51 year old woman exhibiting problems with her short term memory. Over time she exhibited more of the features of what we regard as Alzheimer's disease and, after she died, she was found to have evidence of the pathological features of this condition - namely plaques, tangles and atrophy or loss and shrinkage of parts of the brain. We'll discover more about plaques and tangles later in this chapter.

As doctors, we like to think we are a bit, well, sciencey. That's why we use the term doctor. It's really just a convention as our medical degrees, at least in the UK, aren't doctorates. I'm not an MD or PhD. I digress. Surgeons in the UK call themselves Mr or Miss, something to do with the times when they were barbers, apparently. I've met a lot of surgeons, but I'm not sure I'd want any of them giving me a short back and sides. They can whip out my appendix if they like.

Anyway, we still like to feel that we have one foot in science, even if as a family doctor I spend most of my day dealing with more 'social' problems, such as housing or relationship problems. Occasionally even arranging food parcels. That and clearing printer jams. We like things we can see, diagnoses we can make by chopping things up, sending off tests, or looking at things under the microscope.

Alois Alzheimer noticed what we now take for granted as hallmark, cardinal features of Alzheimer's disease. Except back then he might not have had a name for it. He noticed things called neurofibrillary tangles and amyloid plaques. Other features we tend to see are synaptic degradation (loss of the bits at the ends of nerves) and loss of neurons in the hippocampus. The hippocampus (or hippocampi as we have two, one on each side) is really important in the movement of memories from short to long term memory.

Synapses are at the ends of nerves. They are filled with chemicals called neurotransmitters that can pass the signal onto the next part of the nerve. If these synapses don't work as well, less of the neurotransmitter is available and the signal can't be passed on quite as well. It's a bit like a relay race but, in this case, the runner drops the baton.

We also see loss of neurons in the hippocampus. Neurons are nerve cells (you've probably gathered that by now) and the hippocampus is a part of the brain responsible for an awful lot of rather important things. Much like the rest of the brain. It's a tiny structure, located deep within the brain, and communicates with a whole host of other areas. There are a lot of pathways in and out of the hippocampus. Damage to this area, such as occurs in Alzheimer's, types of stroke and even schizophrenia and severe depression, causes problems with memory formation. Depending on what part is damaged, we might notice problems with remembering the past, or creating new memories. We used to think that we were born with all the brain cells we will ever have, but we know this to be untrue. New cells are made in the hippocampus throughout life. It's a busy little part of the brain. It's this part of the brain that tends to take the greatest clobbering in Alzheimer's disease. This explains why many people explain to me that either they or their loved ones 'can remember the past like it was yesterday, but can't remember what I've just said'. That part of the brain has a lot to answer for.

We've discussed how brilliant brains are and what important bits tend to stop working as well in Alzheimer's, but the question remains: what causes Alzheimer's disease?

We've mentioned structures called plaques and tangles. When we look at a brain of someone with dementia (traditionally once they are finished with it) we can find things called amyloid plaques. These are clumps of something called amyloid-beta (Aβ). These plaques are regarded as features of Alzheimer's disease, but are present in many people long before the disease manifests itself in terms of signs and symptoms. Most people, if not all, who pass the age of 100 have plaques and tangles, and up to about 90 per cent of people at this age have some form of memory problem.

The changes that lead up to a diagnosis of Alzheimer's disease, be it those seen under a microscope or seen in our loved ones or my patients, tend to develop gradually, starting years if not decades before the disease becomes apparent. For many, it may not be that significant, at least not initially. It does make you worry though. The everyday memory lapses that we all encounter, the 'tip of the tongue' phenomenon, the odd word finding problem; could they be the start of something more serious? I sincerely hope not, but only time will tell.

Once Alzheimer's disease sets in, most people tend to live with the condition for anywhere up to a decade. As this is a disease of later life, it doesn't necessarily mean that Alzheimer's disease is life limiting per se, but it certainly has the potential to be quality of life limiting in many cases (at least to the casual observer).

Most cases of Alzheimer's are 'just one of those things'. Sporadic, a case of bad luck or fate? As mentioned, it occurs later in life, but there are a number of risk factors. Some are genetic - there's not much we can do about those, apart from blame our parents. Others are more within our control, to some extent at least. We mentioned previously that Alzheimer's disease is caused, in part, by the development of plaques and tangles. Aβ plaques and neurofibrillary tangles. These form in many of us throughout life, but it is failure to clear them that seems to cause the problem. Traditionally, the diagnosis is made long after symptoms become apparent, perhaps due to a desire not to face up to the potential diagnosis, or the perception that 'I'm alright'. There are techniques available to look for the Aβ plaques, such as specialized types of imaging (positron emission tomography (PET)) but, in reality, the diagnosis is made on the basis of what you tell us, some blood tests and a memory test (see Chapter 4). I've personally not met anyone so far who has had a PET scan for dementia, so I suspect this very much lies within the realms of research.

Alzheimer's is a progressive condition, in as much as it slowly, over time, gets worse. Exactly how severe, and how quickly, is highly individual. These Aβ plaques, the ones that our body can't get rid of, accumulate in the spaces between the cells. They also develop in the walls of our blood vessels. Neurofibrillary tangles are found inside the cells, an accumulation of a protein called tau. The plaques are outside the cells, and tangles are inside.

The plaques are caused by a splitting of a precursor protein, called Amyloid Precursor Protein. Science is nothing if not descriptive. Problems with genes, namely PSEN 1 (presenilin 1) and PSEN 2 (presenilin 2) contribute to the production of amyloid plaques. As do mutations in the genes for Amyloid Precursor Protein.

Most people who are diagnosed with Alzheimer's are in their late seventies or early eighties. For some reason it seems to be more common in women than men. As to why, I'm uncertain. There is a body of evidence that suggests that nerve cells in the hippocampus tend to develop more strongly in the presence of oestrogen (the main female hormone), which makes me wonder if Alzheimer's is more common in women after the menopause, at which point their oestrogen levels are low. Also, men tend to die a little sooner than women, around about five years or so, in which case there are usually more elderly women than there are elderly men. Something like that anyway.

We mentioned earlier about risk factors. Some things are genetic, some are potentially under our control. It appears that diabetes, high blood pressure in mid-life, being obese, physically inactive, depressed, a smoker and with relatively low educational attainment are all risk factors. Some of these things are definitely in our control.

We can lose weight. It might not be easy once you've packed it on, but it is possible. Physical activity is within everyone's reach. The best form of exercise is the one we are doing. I can't really think of many people that I wouldn't recommend physical activity to. Depression is a medical problem in itself, eminently treatable and most people get better, be it with medications, talking therapy or a combination of the two. Smoking? No excuse for it. Just stop. You can get plenty of help to stop smoking. Regarding education, well, we know that people with a high intellectual reserve, basically a good degree of educational ability, tend to deteriorate a little more slowly. Perhaps look at it as a bucket with a leak. If you start with more water in it, it takes longer to empty. I'm not certain how you might improve this, apart from becoming a relentless autodidact. Learn things, lots of things, and keep doing it until you can't.

It's interesting (well, it is to me) that these things are, to a large degree, very similar to the risk factors for heart disease and stroke. Perhaps it makes sense that what's good for the heart should be good for the brain too.

Just how important each of those risk factors is, who can say? But bringing these things into check, making simple changes, will help your general health and wellbeing, and *might* just help prevent cognitive decline later in life, or at the very least reduce the impact that Alzheimer's might have.

There are a few genetic problems that appear to contribute to the development of Alzheimer's disease. One rare form, which starts much younger, has been shown to be due to a number of genetic defects, which ultimately hasten the development of these amyloid plaques and make it hard for the brain to clear them. For instance, early onset inherited Alzheimer's disease has been linked to mutations in a number of genes, including PSEN1 and PSEN2. These are, perhaps aptly called, presenilin genes. Most mutations lead to an overproduction of the Aβ amyloid plaques. Defects in genes called APOE genes (involved in chemical pathways that handle fats) seem to be linked to the development of Alzheimer's disease. There are a number of subtypes, but it is APOE4 that appears to confer the greatest risk. A person carrying one copy of the faulty gene has three times the risk of developing Alzheimer's, but if they carry both there's 12 times the risk. As with all genetic tests the question is: would you want to find out if you carried the defective gene?

3
Other types of dementia

As with much of the amazing thing that is the human body, there are a myriad of ways it can go wrong. Most of the time we work. Mostly. We might take it for granted until bits of it stop working, drop off or point in the wrong direction. Much like the rest of us, there are a substantial number of ways the brain can become faulty. There are quite a large number of different types of dementia, and we'll run through them in this chapter. Safe to say, you'll probably notice quite a bit in common.

I won't go into too much detail, just enough to give an idea about what the condition is and what we might notice in ourselves or loved ones if we suspect some form of dementia. More information about treatment and investigations will come later. A lot of investigations for many of the different types of dementia are not unique to the discovery of a specific disease type. We have a finite number of treatments, almost irrespective of what kind of dementia we might be dealing with.

First up, and in no particular order, vascular dementia.

Vascular dementia

The word 'vascular' pertains to the blood supply. Much as we get cardiovascular disease (a disease of the blood supply to the heart and the heart itself), we can also get cerebrovascular disease. This is a disease of the blood supply to the brain. Vascular cognitive decline and vascular dementia are brought about by a reduction in blood flow to the brain.

Strictly speaking, 'pure' vascular dementia, which is dementia solely due to a lack of blood to the brain, is rare. In reality, most people have 'mixed dementia' when their brains are studied at post-mortem. This means that there are signs of dementia due to Alzheimer's disease, mainly the plaques and tangles, as well as evidence that the blood supply to parts of the brain has been poor or reduced.

We tend to diagnose vascular dementia quite a bit, particularly if someone we see has had strokes that lead up to their cognitive difficulties but, in reality, most dementia is probably a mixture of the two. Life is very rarely black and white, and neither is medicine.

We tend to treat vascular dementia in terms of the risk factors for it. Namely treating blood pressure, diabetes, and lowering cholesterol. Whether this makes a difference is less clear, particularly when the condition really only makes itself known after an event like a stroke (called a cerebrovascular accident) or a mini-stroke (transient ischaemic attack).

The spectrum of vascular cognitive impairment ranges from mild decline to severe dementia. We might notice that someone becomes a bit mentally slower. They might struggle with planning and organizing, or they may develop behavioural problems. People might notice problems with short term memory, or develop psychological problems such as anxiety or depression, or lose interest in their everyday activities. As you'll discover, while the actual diagnoses may differ, there's a fair amount of overlap in terms of symptoms.

When a clinician examines a patient, they might expect to find a number of clinical signs. These are clues that point us towards the possible diagnosis. In the days before laboratory investigations and medical imaging, all we had to go on was what someone said and what we find when we look at them. Let us not underestimate the value of looking closely and listening carefully. I think this is probably pretty good advice for life in general, but I digress.

We tend to see abnormal reflexes. Reflexes are pathways of nerves that cause us to respond without thinking. They might be different on either side of the body. There might be speech problems, which we in the trade refer to as dysarthria; Problems forming words or unclear speech. There may be something called Parkinsonism. Parkinsonism is what we call clinical findings that look a bit like Parkinson's but aren't actually caused by Parkinson's disease. Namely a tremor, a shuffling way of walking, a face that lacks expression. We might notice stiffness of the limbs, called rigidity. The patient or loved one might complain of urinary incontinence. What we notice and how the problems manifest themselves depend very much on what parts of the brain are affected.

While pure vascular dementia is rare, probably about one in ten cases of dementia as a whole, as many as three quarters of patients with dementia may have signs of vascular disease in their brains when inspected at post-mortem. It just goes to show that diagnosis is, at the very best, a highly educated estimate of what is really going on in a body. It isn't possible to be 100 per cent certain of anything. Again, that's probably more a life lesson than a pearl of clinical wisdom.

Most vascular dementia diagnoses are probably 'mixed dementia', so will likely have an element somewhat like Alzheimer's disease in terms of symptoms, prognosis and, ultimately, disease changes in the brain. Exactly what proportion of the condition is due to what process, i.e. vascular disease versus Alzheimer's, is hard to define.

In terms of making a diagnosis, we might well term the condition vascular dementia if there has been some form of cerebrovascular event prior to the development of cognitive impairment. Namely a stroke, or series of mini-strokes. The result could be anything from mild symptoms to full blown dementia. I do wonder how many people have a degree of cerebrovascular disease without even noticing.

Vascular dementia is probably the second most common dementia in terms of diagnoses. Anywhere from one sixth to one third of people with dementia are thought to have vascular dementia. It tends to be more common the older we get, especially after the age of 80. It tends to be life shortening, more so than Alzheimer's, and this might be due to the other problems that are associated with vascular disease in general, such as heart disease. Survival after a diagnosis of vascular dementia tends to be three to five years, and for Alzheimer's around seven to ten years.

There are a number of risk factors that might increase the chances of developing vascular dementia. Perhaps unsurprisingly, having a stroke increases the risk of developing vascular dementia and, as survival from stroke is improving, we might well see more of this. However, faster treatment of stroke means that less of the brain is affected by a reduction in blood flow, meaning less of a deficit after recovery. We are also getting better at reducing the risk of stroke by treating high cholesterol and blood pressure, and we know that doing this causes a decline in the risk of developing stroke. Other factors influencing the development of vascular dementia include being overweight or obese, having diabetes, and suffering from a heart rhythm disturbance called atrial fibrillation. Atrial fibrillation is where the top chambers of the heart, known as the atria, beat in a poorly controlled fashion. Instead of a regular 'buh-dum, buh-dum' of the heartbeat, think more random free form jazz at a high tempo. The heart rate is poorly coordinated, usually fast, and can predispose to the clotting of blood in the upper chamber of the heart. These clots can fling off into the circulation, lodge in the brain and cause a stroke. And what do strokes make? Vascular dementia, at least in some cases. So atrial fibrillation is not great (but this stroke risk can be reduced using anticoagulants).

There are a number of other risk factors, in addition to those named above. Being female seems to increase the risk, as does low educational attainment, low socio-economic class, high blood pressure, past heart disease, stroke, high cholesterol, depression, smoking and low physical activity. We are probably familiar with the health messages about having a healthy heart. Well, the same can be said for the brain, at least in terms of risk of vascular dementia. So stop smoking, get some exercise, lose some weight and lower your blood pressure.

You can see that some of these risk factors can be adjusted. Namely the lifestyle issues. It's less easy, of course, to prevent being depressed - it's not like depression is a lifestyle choice.

There are a number of processes occurring that lead to the development of vascular dementia. Areas of the brain where the blood has stopped flowing are called infarcts. You can get an infarct anywhere. You might have heard of the term 'myocardial infarct', or MI. That's where the heart muscle dies off due to lack of blood supply. Well, in this case it's the brain that gets infarcted. You might see large infarcts, small ones, little ones called lacunar infarcts (which means 'lake' infarcts), microinfarcts, as well as narrowing of the arteries, and damage to blood vessel walls. However, by the time we notice symptoms, the exact mechanism is probably pretty academic. That said, knowing a little about the process can help us understand why we end up having the treatment we do when a disease is diagnosed.

If a bit of brain is infarcted then it doesn't work, at least not as well as it did. The number, location and size of infarct tends to affect the likelihood of cognitive impairment. Multiple infarcts, large infarcts and infarcts in areas of the cerebral cortex tend to increase the chance of developing vascular dementia. Areas of the brain affected tend to become inflamed initially. Inflammation is the way the body fixes itself, but inflammation doesn't always help. You might notice this when we get a scratch or a cut. The affected area becomes inflamed, which might help it heal, but it doesn't tend to work very well in the process.

In terms of making a diagnosis, I've touched on how we might come to the conclusion earlier. But, in general terms, we expect to see a number of areas of cognition, or brain function, negatively affected. We usually see memory impairment, which is frequently what brings people to see us. Other cognitive deficits are apparent. These might include changes in behaviour, depression or anxiety. Problems with walking, such as a shuffling gait, might become apparent. Diagnosis is usually based on clinical judgement. That's doctor speak for 'what I reckon'. Also, evidence of cognitive impairment on memory tests. The one I tend to use is called the Addenbrooke's Cognitive Examination III (ACE-III). There are a number of investigations available which may help us decide if a person has some form of dementia. Scans might show evidence of vascular disease in the brain. We'll talk more about what to expect in clinic in a later chapter. We usually make the diagnosis if the problems with memory and thinking are noticed after a cerebrovascular event, like a stroke.

Other problems affecting the brain can seem a little like vascular dementia. These include Alzheimer's, dementia with Lewy bodies, frontotemporal dementia, and even depression. As I've said before, there's a big overlap. This makes the potential diagnosis all the more challenging. It's quite difficult to untie all the potential symptoms but, as you'll see in later chapters, treatment often overlaps as much as the potential diagnosis.

The core features of vascular dementia usually include a stepwise deterioration in cognition. Whereas Alzheimer's disease is classically a gradual deterioration, vascular dementia usually gets worse after some form of cerebrovascular event. There is often a temporal association between the stroke/mini-stroke and the decline in memory. The sorts of problems that are noticed tend to be associated with memory, attention, language, visuospatial skills (noticing where things are in space) and something called executive function, which encompasses all the skills we need to operate in the world. We'll talk more about how we go onto diagnose dementia in a later chapter but, in general terms, you can expect a visit to a memory clinic, some blood tests, a brain scan of some form and a special test to look at different areas of cognitive function.

Dementia with Lewy bodies

Dementia with Lewy bodies (DLB) is probably the next most common form of dementia we see. It probably represents about five per cent of all dementia. The Lewy body part of the name refers to small areas noticed within cells under a microscope. Once again, this is usually during a post-mortem. We tend to try to leave people's brains alone while they are alive.

In terms of symptoms, there's a fair amount of overlap between DLB, Parkinson's disease and Parkinson's disease dementia, which makes the diagnosis a little less straightforward. There's a trend here in as much as a clinical diagnosis is dependent on what information is available to us and the signs and symptoms a person exhibits. There are only so many ways our body can show us that it isn't working that well.

DLB affects both cognitive function - thinking, performing actions, etc., as well as movement, which is why there appears to be an overlap in terms of features with Parkinson's disease. We might notice problems with attention, visuospatial skills and, once again, executive function. Basically thinking, doing, initiating and finishing tasks. The sort of everyday stuff we take for granted. People tend to struggle with fluency of speech and visual perception. People may notice difficulties in solving problems. We also notice other problems such as visual hallucinations, sleeping problems and the features of Parkinsonism, such as a shuffling gait, increased muscle rigidity and tremor, particularly at rest. Other features may lend themselves to the diagnosis, such as excessive daytime sleepiness or absence of smell. (It must be said that there are lots of causes of poor smell and being sleepy in the day. I'm not sure I've felt awake in the day since I qualified as a doctor, and even less so since my children arrived.) The features I tend to look for are shuffling, rigidity, cognitive problems and hallucinations. That would probably be enough for me to make the diagnosis. We'll talk more about treatment in a later chapter.

Parkinson's disease dementia

In terms of symptoms, there is a fair bit of overlap between Parkinson's disease dementia and dementia with Lewy bodies. In the case of Parkinson's disease, the problems we see with movement tend to occur first, then the memory problems occur. There's a general reduction in cognitive abilities, and it's usually enough to have a noticeable impact on the activities of daily life. Memory starts to suffer, as does carrying out daily activities such as personal care, washing, cooking and cleaning. Movements become slower and harder to perform. The key thing to remember is this occurs in the context of established, already diagnosed Parkinson's disease. Parkinson's is traditionally regarded as a movement disorder, with rigid/stiff limbs, a tremor, slower movements and a drop in blood pressure on standing. While not everyone with Parkinson's disease will get dementia, having Parkinson's increases the risk of developing dementia in general, compared to those without the condition.

While Parkinson's disease can be largely regarded as a disease primarily affecting movement, memory disturbances and problems with thinking can also occur. Parkinson's disease is caused by a progressive reduction in dopamine producing nerve cells in a part of the brain called the basal ganglia. It isn't apparent clinically until over half of the nerves that produce this neurotransmitter have disappeared. We mentioned earlier some of the features of Parkinson's disease, namely slow movements, tremor and limb rigidity. There's a crossover with DLB, but in Parkinson's disease dementia, the movement disorder comes first, in Lewy body it's the cognitive problems that present sooner.

Parkinson's disease is pretty common, and about 140,000 people live in the UK with Parkinson's disease at present. It's more common the older we get, and is more common in men than in women. It's slowly progressive and generally reduces life expectancy. In addition to memory impairment, people with Parkinson's disease can experience depression, anxiety, panic attacks, loss of interest in their usual activities, not to mention dementia.

About one third of people with Parkinson's disease dementia have some form of cognitive impairment at the time of diagnosis. They tend to struggle with concentration, visuospatial problems, excessive daytime sleepiness, visual hallucinations and delusions.

Frontotemporal dementia

The next type of dementia I want to talk about is called Frontotemporal dementia (FTD). I must admit, FTD isn't something I've seen much of. Or at least, it isn't something I've recognized in a patient until their dementia is pretty well advanced. It really best describes a group of conditions that cause atrophy, or shrinkage of parts of the frontal or temporal lobes of the brain, and sometimes both. Hence the name.

FTD tends to affect behaviour or language, causing changes in behaviour or difficulties with either producing speech or understanding it. As with the other types of dementia touched upon so far, there's a bit of an overlap in terms of symptoms, particularly with Parkinson's disease and motor neurone disease (MND). FTD tends to present earlier than Alzheimer's in general, namely in mid-life. Initially, there may be no problems with memory, orientation in space and time or general intelligence and cognitive function. The behavioural variant might present with problems akin to depression, anxiety or psychosis and, because FTD isn't that common but mental illness is, we might diagnose a patient with depression and start treating it, rather than expect FTD. Early problems with language might be put down to depression or anxiety, and thus dismissed as early FTD. You can see that in the early stages, making a diagnosis is somewhat challenging.

In terms of language, you might notice problems with long words, or the development of a speech impediment such as a stutter. Problems with grammar or recall of specialized jargon usually used in a job or hobby might start to emerge. These symptoms are pretty general, so it's no wonder such a condition might go undiagnosed or unrecognized initially.

In terms of behaviour, we might notice problems developing with interpersonal relationships, emotional responses, initiating and carrying out everyday tasks, or developing quite marked changes in behaviour (such as becoming disinhibited, losing interest in previously enjoyable activities, developing obsessions and ritualistic behaviour). You can see that these changes could easily be put down to mental illness, a 'mid-life crisis' or 'nervous breakdown'.

Other features noticed in the behavioural variant include changes in food preferences, social behaviours, humour, developing obsessional hobbies, spontaneous, distractible and impulsive behaviours, and I've even heard of increased mid-life religiosity.

In the speech-based variants we might notice problems with the understanding of speech, particularly formerly recognizable words. Speech becomes less fluent, and it's harder to convey views and opinions. Meanings of words might get lost. There might be difficulty remembering names, understanding the meanings of words, particularly affecting specialized knowledge. Loss of recognition of normally familiar faces may occur. I've seen this on a number of occasions, and once looked after someone who could recognize her husband in wedding pictures, partly because she was in them too, but very much unable to recognize him in the flesh. This caused some considerable distress for all concerned. Medically fascinating, but a complete nightmare for those affected.

As with other dementias, there's an overlap in symptoms with other conditions. These include rarer neuro-degenerative conditions such as corticobasal syndrome and supranuclear palsy, and even motor neurone disease with intercurrent frontotemporal dementia. We'll touch on these less commonly encountered conditions later. FTD, like Alzheimer's disease, is another condition caused by the build up of abnormal proteins in the brain, albeit different ones to those seen in Alzheimer's disease. There's a genetic element to it too, with some cases of FTD being hereditary to some degree. These are due to specific genetic defects. In terms of prognosis, FTD progresses steadily, with a reduction in the ability of the person to carry out everyday activities. Problems occur with thinking, social skills, with disability developing and many needing long term residential care in time. For some people, this can take as few as a few years, for others the time scale may be as much as a decade or so. FTD can cause significant behavioural problems (including loss of interest in life), problems swallowing, wandering off, challenging behaviours, urinary incontinence and even mutism. People can just stop speaking. Understandably this can cause significant stress on the part of the carers, be they professional or informal family carers.

Mild cognitive impairment

Mild cognitive impairment is pretty self-explanatory. It's basically memory problems sufficient to notice, but not quite enough to cause problems. Much like the other conditions mentioned previously, we tend to notice problems with language, memory, thinking skills and judgement. It tends to be worse than expected for age, but not severe enough to be called dementia. Depending on your source of statistics, as many as one fifth of people over the age of 65 are thought to have mild cognitive impairment. In general, it's more common the older we get, with a greater proportion of people being affected over the age of 80 than in younger age brackets. For some, mild cognitive impairment can be an early indicator of Alzheimer's disease, but a diagnosis of mild cognitive impairment doesn't mean that developing Alzheimer's is a given. While there's no specific treatment for mild cognitive impairment, there are a number of risk factors and addressing these might help prevent it. Much like vascular dementia, controlling blood pressure, diabetes, cholesterol, and giving up smoking could help prevent the development of mild cognitive impairment.

In many cases, mild cognitive impairment could be so mild that it's hardly noticed. This is particularly the case as the ability to carry out every day activities is rarely impaired.

Around 30 to 50 per cent of those diagnosed with mild cognitive impairment will go on to develop some form of dementia within a decade of noticing symptoms, but it's important to state that a significant proportion of people won't go on to be afflicted.

A proportion of causes of mild cognitive impairment could be down to reversible causes. When we refer people onto memory clinic, we usually do a full set of blood tests to look for these potentially reversible causes. These include an underactive thyroid gland and low vitamin B12 levels. Other potential causes (that, in fairness, we won't pick up with a blood test) include raised pressure in the brain or something called a chronic subdural haematoma. These occur when blood leaks beneath one of the coatings of the brain (called the dura), usually after a minor head injury. It can cause a gradual onset cognitive impairment and is usually detected with careful history taking and some form of head scan.

Other conditions that can present in later life include poor memory, common psychological conditions (such as anxiety, depression and stress), underlying infections, medication side effects, biochemical abnormalities, and even constipation.

Posterior cortical atrophy

I'm not sure I've ever seen this. Not overtly anyway. This is a rare form of progressive dementia affecting the back (posterior) of the brain. It has features similar to Alzheimer's from a pathological point of view, namely plaques and tangles, but mainly affects vision, and could present with problems in spelling, writing and mathematics skills. The back of the brain, the occipital lobe, is what we use to see. We might think we see with the eyes but, without a functioning visual cortex, we are blind. We can have perfect eyes but still be blind if the back of the brain isn't working.

Given that the business end of vision starts to play up, many people with Posterior cortical atrophy (PCA) might present to their optician, only to be told their eyes are in good health. We might notice problems with recognition, visuospatial awareness or judgement when driving (such as the speed of other cars, distances, or seeing things as moving when they are, in fact, still). Colour vision might be affected, and there might be problems tolerating bright light. Problems with writing may occur, and there may be problems with activities of daily living such as getting dressed or washing.

PCA tends to become apparent at a younger age than Alzheimer's disease, starting as young as the mid-fifties. Symptoms are often subtle and the list above is by no means exhaustive. There are grades of severity, from very early PCA with no apparent features to a quite advanced disease, causing considerable impact on cognition, ability to perform everyday activities, memory impairment and visual problems to the point of blindness.

Mixed dementia

We mentioned earlier that, in reality, most dementia is probably mixed to some degree, and usually a mixture of Alzheimer's and vascular dementia. This isn't always the case as we tend to find combinations of other dementias too. Symptoms in part depend on the pathological processes in the brain, with mixtures of symptoms depending on which areas of the brain are affected and by what condition. It tends to be more common in those in their mid-seventies onwards, with treatment tailored to the dominant set of symptoms.

Young onset dementia

This is dementia that is apparent before the age of 65. To some extent this is a relatively arbitrary cut off point but, as most dementia we see is at older age ranges, it probably isn't unreasonable. It tends to make up about five per cent of cases of dementia, and can have a wide range of causes. Mostly, people experience problems with memory, movement, coordination and balance. There's an increased hereditary nature in young onset dementia, with as many as one in ten people having a familial form.

Causes, much as for older age groups, include Alzheimer's; underlying Down's syndrome or learning difficulties; vascular causes, including a genetic form of vascular dementia called CADASIL (cerebral autosomal dominant arteriopathy with subcortical infarcts and leukoencephalopathy); frontotemporal dementia; dementia with Lewy bodies and alcohol. Rarer forms include Huntington's disease (a genetically inherited condition that causes problems with movement and cognition), progressive supranuclear palsy, corticobasal degeneration, and even rarer metabolic conditions such as Tay-Sachs disease, Gaucher's and Niemann-Pick's disease. I won't be discussing these to any great extent as they are incredibly rare, at least by comparison to conditions such as Alzheimer's disease.

Creutzfeldt-Jakob disease (CJD)

There are three types of CJD, namely sporadic, inherited and iatrogenic/new variant CJD. CJD is a prion disease. Prions are proteins that can cause infection and subsequent degeneration of a person's brain. They are very rare indeed. I think I've seen perhaps one case in my whole career to date. Most are sporadic, a case of bad luck with a mutation occurring in one of our own prion proteins causing the condition. This is not transmissible. Hereditary CJD tends to occur in family clusters but is pretty rare. Finally, iatrogenic/variant CJD cases are even rarer still. Iatrogenic means a problem is caused by the people looking after you, namely doctors. It can be transmitted during neurosurgery, via tissue grafts or from hormone treatments extracted from cadavers (also known as dead people), particularly the pituitary gland.

Variant CJD is linked to the prevalence of Bovine Spongiform Encephalopathy which was a problem in the late 1980s in cattle. It was thought at one point that we would all get it, due to eating infected meat during this time. By now we were meant to be expecting a tidal wave of CJD caused by infected burgers, but this remains to be seen. I'm not expecting to see any cases of this in my career.

Symptoms tend to include a rapidly progressive degenerative condition affecting the brain, with problems with personality change, visual impairment, jerking of the limbs, blindness, loss of movement, loss of voice and progressive memory loss. It sounds truly horrific, and I'm glad there aren't many cases of this.

The iatrogenic/transmissible form tends to be caused by exposure to brain tissue and spinal cord fluid of infected persons, such as pituitary growth hormone injections, corneal transplants, and meat that was tainted with neural tissue. In other words, burgers full of bits of brain and spinal cord. It certainly makes the case for vegetarianism all the more compelling. I don't think anyone's ever got seriously ill from a carrot...

Alcoholic dementia

Alcohol is, on the whole, not good for you. I used to like a drink but now I've become one of those boring people who don't drink and tells everyone how great it is to be teetotal. Medical school was a bit of a house-red-coloured blur. The older I get, the less I enjoy alcohol and the more I enjoy waking up with a clear head, not wanting to be sick, and being able to remember the night before. There probably isn't such a thing as a safe level of alcohol, at least the more we know about it.

Alcohol can cause dementia, and I've seen this a fair bit. No disease is nice to witness or suffer from, or at least no disease I've either experienced myself or treated in others. Alcoholic dementia is a cruel, brutal waste of life and utterly preventable. I've seen people destroyed by alcohol, and not just them but the lives of those they love. Except, for some, the love of the grain or grape can be greater than that of those around them.

In essence, alcohol-related brain damage (including alcoholic dementia) is caused by long term alcohol misuse and vitamin deficiency. It tends to affect those from their forties upwards, and is the result of long term, regular alcohol excess. Stopping the alcohol can lead to a partial recovery and, in some, a complete recovery. It could prevent worsening of already established alcohol-related brain damage.

Alcohol is toxic to the brain. Excessive alcohol can cause a lack of thiamine in the body. Thiamine is a B vitamin, important for the production of energy in the body and brain, as well as nerve cell function. Thiamine deficiency tends to occur in the context of a poor diet and reduced absorption. Hardcore drinkers traditionally forgo food for alcohol, compounding the problem. Being under the influence a lot of the time predisposes us to falls, and repeated low level brain injury might well add to the development of brain damage. Alcohol affects our judgement, and leads to poor decisions. Heavy drinkers also tend to have a number of other risk factors including vascular disease, high blood pressure, high cholesterol, an increased risk of stroke and heart disease.

The mainstay of treatment is prevention, and to address the risk factors. About one in 200 people have alcohol-related brain damage of some form. That's half a per cent. That's loads of people. By the time we reach those with alcohol dependence, this figure rises to one in three. A third of all people with alcohol dependence have some form of brain damage as a result. It affects younger people, tends to be more common in men (and in women in poorer communities), but occurs in women at a younger age than men.

Chronic alcohol misuse can lead to a phenomenon known as Wernicke's encephalopathy, caused by an abrupt cessation of alcohol use in those with a degree of alcohol dependence. People get confused, agitated, with involuntary jerking movements, poor balance and unsteadiness. Left untreated it can develop into Korsakoff's psychosis, which leads to irreparable damage to the brain.

Alcoholic dementia has a range of symptoms, depending on the part of the brain that is affected. We might notice poor decision making and organizational skills, challenges with financial situations, problems with emotion, poor planning skills, problems with attention, and behavioural inhibition.

Delirium tremens is an acute reaction occurring in someone who has had excessive alcohol, long term, and it can be fatal. It involves anxiety, restlessness, tremors, excessive sweating, disorientation, hallucination and an intense feeling of fear. It tends to occur within a few days of stopping alcohol completely in the context of alcohol dependence, but is easily treated providing it is recognized. Long term alcohol use can also cause significant problems with the liver, ultimately leading to cirrhosis or irreversible scarring and shrinkage. This can lead to a condition called hepatic encephalopathy. If the liver isn't doing its job, neurotoxic compounds can build up in the brain causing confusion and cognitive deficits.

Corticobasal degeneration

This is a rare type of dementia, and subsequently something your local family doctor will see very rarely in their career, if at all. It's a pretty nasty condition, but no form of dementia seems like a great deal of fun. Symptoms vary between individuals, and not everyone gets all the symptoms. Those affected tend to get progressive stiffness, are unable to make purposeful movements with the affected limb(s) and it gets progressively worse over time. It tends to affect skilful, coordinated movements, and may get noticed when someone struggles to carry out everyday tasks such as buttoning a shirt or combing their hair.

Symptoms usually start on one side of the body and, over time, progress to affect both sides of the body (and, by definition, the brain). We might notice tremors, slowness of movement or lack of it, jerking of the limbs, problems speaking and contractures of the limbs where they are locked in a flexed position. There may be memory loss, a loss of inhibitions and interest, poor attention or obsessive behaviours. Over time, the ability to communicate is diminished, as well as increasing disability, with the sufferer becoming bedridden. It is a life limiting condition.

The causes of corticobasal degeneration are unknown. Areas of the brain lose tissue and, as I said before, if it's missing it isn't doing its job. Areas of the brain atrophy or shrink, with the symptoms displayed dependent on which parts of the brain are gradually disappearing.

It tends to affect men and women equally, with symptoms developing in people in their fifties onwards. It's virtually unheard of in people under 40, and affects around 0.00005 per cent of the population. That's about five in 100,000. Like I say, it's rather rare. As a result, we might not think of it as a diagnosis, misdiagnose it as another form of dementia or neuro-degenerative condition, or not even think of it at all.

HIV-related cognitive impairment

This is another rare form of dementia that we don't see very often in family medicine. It causes fairly mild problems in thinking, memory and reasoning and, as such, might go unnoticed, or put down to other issues. Before the advent of antiretroviral medications, it was seen in between a fifth and a third of people with advanced HIV. Now, it's seen in fewer than two per cent of cases. It tends to show itself with problems with short term memory, cognitive slowing, concentration problems, decision making, occasional unsteadiness or mood problems. I could quite easily diagnose it as depression, which is massively more common.

Huntington's disease

Huntington's disease is a rare condition, caused by a hereditary genetic mutation that means if you've got the mutation, you'll have the disease, and you'll have passed in on to subsequent generations. It presents with problems with thinking, movement and behaviour, and tends to become apparent in people in their thirties onwards. It is a progressive condition, with movement problems coming first, followed by cognitive problems and, finally, behavioural challenges. It's caused by a faulty gene on chromosome 4. The gene encodes for a protein called Huntingtin, and faults in the gene cause damage to the neurons prior to birth. Each child of a parent carrying the gene has a 50:50 chance of inheriting the gene. There is a genetic test for it, but the question is, would you want to find out? This is a very real problem affecting those with family members with Huntington's disease. It can even impact on the decision of whether to have a family in the first place. Natural conception brings with it potential risks of transmission of the condition, which may lead affected couples to consider fertility treatment and pre-implantation genetic diagnosis.

In the past, Huntington's disease used to be called Huntington's chorea, and chorea means dance. Movement problems (such as problems with dexterity), slurred speech, problems with balance, recurrent falls and swallowing problems occur. Over time, the limbs become more rigid and stiff. Cognitive problems include slowing of thoughts, processing of information, problems initiating simple tasks and organizational skills. The more negative effects that develop, the greater the negative effect on quality of life. Problems with mental health such as depression and anxiety may occur, which is pretty understandable given the nature of the condition. Huntington's is progressive and life limiting, taking its toll on the patient and their loved ones.

Dementia in multiple sclerosis

Multiple sclerosis (MS) is a condition whereby the outer coating of nerves, called myelin, becomes lost. A proportion of people with MS go on to develop problems with memory and thinking. It's thought that almost half of all people with MS develop such problems. It can cause poor memory, slower thinking, problems with complex tasks, problems with executive function (planning, etc.), and problems with visuospatial skills.

There's a marked overlap, at least in terms of symptoms, with many types of dementia. There are a number of different classifications of MS, but secondary progressive MS tends to be associated with worse cognitive function than others. Short-term memory is particularly affected, but there can also be problems with language as well. People may struggle with recall, attention and concentration. They might notice problems with problem solving, word finding, orientation in space, and general everyday functioning. This is on top of the physical problems that MS tends to cause.

Niemann-Pick disease type C

This is a super rare progressive genetic disorder, which causes problems with the way the body transports fatty substances, such as cholesterol, inside cells. I think I might have seen this once when in training, on a metabolic unit specializing in super rare disorders of metabolism. I can't imagine I'll ever see it again. As a GP or family doctor, we often tell people that their cholesterol is too high. Granted, high cholesterol is a risk factor for heart disease and stroke, but it is important to have some, and for it to be handled by the body in the proper fashion.

Most cases are discovered at childhood, and can vary in fashion from a rapidly fatal disorder to a late onset, slowly progressive disease that tends to remain undiagnosed until late in childhood. It's caused by mutations of genes called NPC1 and NPC2. It tends to occur equally in men and women, but only occurs about once in every 100,000 live births. Symptoms include problems swallowing, seizures, problems with muscle tone, lung disease, learning disorders, a whole raft of psychological problems, movement problems, sleep disorders, falls, developmental delay, hearing loss, and problems with eye movements. This list is by no means exhaustive but with such a varied set of symptoms, some milder forms may be missed in terms of diagnosis, or wrongly labelled as a different condition.

Normal pressure hydrocephalus

This is another rare form of dementia. It is recognized by these characteristics: problems with gait, large cerebral ventricles (fluid-filled spaces within the brain) and no other apparent cause. Consequently, it's a diagnosis of exclusion to some extent. Hydrocephalus is a condition whereby there's too much fluid within the brain. This usually causes a build up in pressure within the brain and the ventricles, these fluid-filled areas within the brain, are seen to expand in the context of raised pressure within the brain. However, in the case of normal pressure hydrocephalus, the pressure within the brain of the person is OK. Hence the name: normal pressure hydrocephalus.

In terms of symptoms, we might notice a tremor, rigidity of the limbs, visual hallucinations, difficulty speaking, problems with recognition (such as recognizing things or loved ones), but, if recognized, there tends to be an improvement after shunting. With shunting, a tube is inserted under the skin into the ventricles of the brain and channeled through the body into somewhere the fluid can drain, such as the abdominal cavity. It tends to have a slow onset, usually over the age of forty, with symptoms being present for months before being noticed. Brain scans show enlarged ventricles, these fluid-filled areas of the brain.

Initially we might notice problems with movement, urinary problems and difficulty with thinking, including behavioural problems. Over time the condition develops, with more and more disability and an ultimate need for hands-on care.

Progressive supranuclear palsy

Progressive supranuclear palsy is a rare, progressive condition causing problems with the eyes, movement problems such as unexplained falls, a disturbance of gait, a low mood, problems word finding, executive function, and emotional disturbance. There's a bit of an overlap in terms of Parkinson's disease. There is no known treatment.

Summary

In summary, there are quite a few different types of dementia. Many have symptoms in common, some have more distinguishing features. Some have treatments available (more on that later), some don't. Some present at advanced years, some in relative youth. Some are genetic, many aren't. Some are related to other medical conditions, some are causes of dementia in their own right. Most, if not all are progressive and, in many cases, they lead to life changing consequences. Dementia, almost regardless of the cause, robs us of who we are, of our loved ones and of our futures. Or at least we might perceive that. Dementia does change lives, it can shorten them, but it is what it is. We might not be able to change the hand we're dealt, but we can try to live our best lives despite the diagnosis we might acquire.

Over the next few chapters, we'll find out more about what happens if you suspect an underlying dementia, what treatments are available and how to get help. The thing about dementia is that it is very common. Sure, there are rare forms, but there's a lot of people out there with dementia, you're not alone and there's a lot of help out there. The problem is, if you don't know it's there, you don't go looking. Hopefully, after the next few chapters, you won't have to look much further to get help.

4
What happens in clinic?

How do we get the help we need if we suspect we, or a member of our family, might have Alzheimer's disease (or any other dementia, come to that)? Sometimes it's difficult to know, particularly in the early stages. We can coast along quite nicely, until something happens that uncovers that we've been having problems longer than we care to admit.

We often have suspicions that there might be a problem. We might notice a few more memory failures. We might forget the name of someone we knew once, or not recognize them. We might find ourselves getting lost in usually familiar situations, or not remembering what happens next in a once readily completed task.

More often than not it's our loved ones that notice there's a problem. Often they'll notice our change in demeanour before we do. What we might put down to being stressed or preoccupied actually being the first signs of dementia. Those memory failures we blame on distractions, being the result of pathological changes in our brain. In my experience, it's often the relatives that notice first, and many people I meet who clearly have some form of dementia stubbornly decline to accept it, or are unable to. Like King Canute on the beach, rather than admit that the waves are lapping around our ankles, we try vainly to keep the waves out of reach.

I meet a lot of people who worry about their memory. Sometimes close relatives (usually daughters for some reason, but I'm not sure why) will bring a member of their family to my surgery. We will talk about what problems have been noticed. It might be short term memory problems such as difficulty remembering conversations, or getting lost in previously familiar environments. I hasten to add that these are not the sole diagnostic criteria for dementia. I rarely remember anything my wife tells me, much to her dismay. I can recall random percentages about how common certain diseases are. I have a clear recollection of the Christmas Number 1 in 2004, but I can't remember what my wife has told me ten minutes ago. I also get lost very easily. If I arrive late for a home visit, you'll know why.

On your initial appointment with your doctor, we will most likely arrange a set of blood tests. This is frequently known as a dementia screen. In reality, it's a set of common blood tests that might suggest a physical cause of memory loss. It includes tests such as a full blood count, kidney function tests, liver function tests, as well as other things such as B12 and folic acid level. We'll talk about these tests later.

At the first meeting, if there's enough time, we may carry out a number of cognitive tests. These are questionnaires that look at different areas of thinking and can be used to help detect potential problems. There are a number of tests, including the General Practitioner Assessment of Cognition (GPCOG), the Mini-Mental State Examination (MMSE) and the Addenbrooke's Cognitive Examination (ACE) of which there are a number of variations. The one I tend to use is the GPCOG, which is a very quick and easy screening test. This is a short test of memory and recall and is readily done in the context of a ten minute consultation. It has two parts - one to be filled out by the patient, another to be filled out by someone known to them (delightfully called the 'informant'). If this shows a drop in cognition, the next step is to get the blood tests done to check there are no potentially reversible causes of cognitive impairment.

Many places across the UK have memory clinics. These may be led by a psychiatrist specializing in older people's mental health, a neurologist with an interest in dementia, or an older person's physician (a geriatrician). Appointments are usually longer, and a lot of the initial memory assessment may be carried out by a specialist nurse or mental health practitioner. It is usually here that the longer memory questionnaires are carried out; an example of which is the Addenbrooke's Cognitive Examination. This is also the test I tend to use if I have more time in clinic. Other tests are available.

A further, more detailed discussion may occur, and other issues will be addressed. We'll talk about them in more detail later, but you may discuss areas such as Lasting Power of Attorney, driving, future care requirements, medication options and follow-up plans. As with any illness, a diagnosis of Alzheimer's disease, and dementia in general, has the potential to be life changing. Memory clinic is one of the first steps along the path to greater understanding of the effects of the condition, and how we can live with it, rather than suffer from it.

One of the scariest things about any diagnosis, be it dementia, cancer, in fact any long-term condition, is that there are a fair amount of unknowns. With the advancement of medical science, we know what happens to populations of people with a condition. We might know the average life span after diagnosis, the sorts of problems people might develop, the sorts of treatment we might expect - but we don't really know what will happen to ourselves. Our futures are all unwritten, all uncertain. Having a diagnosis might provide a little less mystery about what tomorrow brings. Only a little. It does, however, allow us to prepare for a future where not all of the decisions we need to make will be made by us.

Anyway, we were discussing what happens in clinic. At some point, you can expect to have a blood test. We look for a series of potentially reversible causes of cognitive impairment. Medical diagnoses are all about patterns. We might get an idea of what's going on from the history, or the story the patient tells us. This helps reveal a little part of the jigsaw image. There is no specific blood test for most causes of dementia, but more tests that slowly reveal a little more detail about what we think is going on. Exactly like an extra piece of a jigsaw. We might not need all of the pieces to recognize what we see in the picture but, in some cases, we will need as many pieces as possible to get a handle on what might be going on. Blood tests are one part of our jigsaw puzzle.

Blood tests are the starting point for investigations of pretty much every condition I deal with. We carry out a whole raft of them, including the following:

- **FBC** - full blood count, looks for anaemia and a raised white cell count which could be a marker of infection.
- **ESR** - erythrocyte sedimentation rate, a nonspecific marker of inflammation. Inflammation is the body's way of fixing things and ESR levels are raised in countless diseases.

- **CRP** - c-reactive protein, a protein made in the liver and raised in inflammatory processes.
- **Thyroid function** - an underactive thyroid can cause cognitive impairment.
- **Calcium levels** - problems with calcium regulation, of which there are many causes, can affect our cognition.
- **Kidney function** - if our kidneys are playing up, it can cause cognitive problems.
- **Vitamin B12 and folic acid** - important vitamins for maintaining brain health.
- **Liver Function and clotting tests** - would help us see if the cognitive impairment is as a result of liver disease.
- **Syphilis screen** - to see if the cognitive impairment is due to syphilis. Apparently, Casanova and Al Capone had it. It's making a bit of a come back in terms of popularity.
- **Copper levels** - a rare liver disease called Wilson's disease can cause copper overload, which can contribute to cognitive impairment.
- **Glucose levels** - diabetes can be an underlying cause of many problems.

Other tests we can use are:

- **Urine tests** - to check for infection. Infections can make people very confused indeed.
- **Chest X-ray** - to look for further infectious foci of cognitive decline.
- **Electrocardiogram (ECG)** - the test that happens when someone wires your chest up to a box of tricks. Helps us see if you've had a heart attack, or if the function of your heart is having a negative impact on your cognition.

It must be said, while many conditions can cause problems with our thinking and mental wellbeing, I don't usually find many. I can't recall the last case I saw of syphilis, for example. We get plenty of people becoming acutely confused in the context of electrolyte abnormalities (the salts that circulate in our blood), but this is usually overlaying a background of someone becoming rapidly confused. The same can be said for infections, not uncommonly the chest or urine being the culprit. People of advanced years can become very confused, very quickly, with relatively mild changes in blood chemistry, or relatively mild infections. That said, I sometimes feel the diagnosis of chest and urinary infections is often overly applied to older people who are confused. I see plenty of people with underactive thyroid glands but, to this day, have not seen anyone so extremely unwell with it that they appear demented. However, if you don't look for it, you won't find it.

More often than not, the blood tests are normal, or mostly normal, or show something else going on that we already knew about or suggests the need for further investigations.

At this point, once anything I can correct in terms of biochemistry or other pathology has been corrected, I'll refer to my local memory assessment clinic. Depending on where you are in the UK, or perhaps even the world, this might be made up of a number of different professionals with an interest in the diagnosis and treatment of dementia. More detailed questions are usually asked in clinic. We'll take a history of problems from the patient themselves, and a history from any loved ones that may also be attending. We'll carry out a physical examination of the patient. Not only are there lots of different types of dementia, but many other conditions that aren't dementia may be apparent. This may include psychological problems such as depression or anxiety; other potential neurological diagnoses (such as MS or motor neurone disease); physical conditions that might cause problems (such as signs of a past stroke); and, finally a cognitive examination, which is one of the many longer form neuropsychological tests, such as the Addenbrooke's Cognitive Examination mentioned previously.

We will tend to ask questions about a person's life to date, such as how long they were in full time education, occupational history, a past medical history as well as any past psychiatric disorders that might lend themselves to aiding diagnosis. A family history, asking about any relatives who might have developed dementia, a social history enquiring about living arrangements, care packages, or if any family members are assisting with care. We will ask about medications as there are plenty of medications that cause cognitive impairment. Opiate medications such as codeine can cause cognitive blunting, drugs used in epilepsy can cause memory difficulties, certain drugs used in the treatment of an overactive bladder can increase the risk of developing dementia. In fact, many of the medications we prescribe can leave us feeling a bit 'knocked off'.

We'll ask loved ones about what they've noticed. Collateral or informant history is often more illuminating in terms of a possible diagnosis than that which is volunteered from the patient. Relatives often notice problems well in advance of the person affected.

We might ask if they appear forgetful, get lost or wander off. We might ask about personality change, ability to carry out daily activities, changes in sleep pattern or mood. This list is, once again, by no means exhaustive, but it might give you some idea about what to expect from memory clinic.

Cognitive testing, of which there are a number available, looks at specific areas of cognitive function. We'll test attention, orientation, memory, language, visuospatial skills, basic motor function (i.e. movement) and overall function. There are at least 12 cognitive scales I've heard of, and probably more besides. Whichever one is used should have been validated and provide repeatable, reliable results to help determine what the underlying diagnosis might be.

The next step is usually to arrange some form of imaging of the brain. Usually a computer tomography (CT) scan or magnetic resonance imaging (MRI). The role of imaging of the brain is to help determine what might be happening and to consider if other processes might be going on in the brain that may be responsible for what our patient is experiencing.

CT scans are probably the first line investigation in terms of imaging of the brain. They are the 'doughnut' scan, as some of my patients have called it. They compose of a ring in which the source of x-rays spins around the patient, who is usually lying on their back facing up. The do involve exposure to ionizing radiation, which can increase the risk of developing cancer if repeatedly exposed. However, the ends usually justify the means. They're good at looking for blood and tumours, which might be responsible for a person's cognitive decline.

MRI is the 'tunnel' scan. The one that involves laying on a platform that sends you through a noisy, banging tube that you're not allowed in if you've got metal in you/on you/inserted into some body part or another. It uses ultra-strong magnetic fields to realign the spin of your protons. This isn't as unpleasant as it sounds as it doesn't involve radiation and, therefore, the increased risk of cancer that CT scans have. MRI scans are better at looking at soft tissues, and the brain is generally pretty soft indeed.

There are more specialized imaging tests, called fluorode-oxyglucose positron emission tomography (FDG-PET) and SPECT (single positron emission computed tomography). In my experience, these are more often seen in the context of research, and isn't something readily available to most family doctors, as far as I am aware.

Once the diagnosis has become all too apparent, the next stage of clinic is to discuss treatments, be they drug related or non-pharmacological, and other areas of practical support and advice. More on that in later chapters.

Going to see your doctor need not be a scary proposition, even if you suspect that you may receive news you don't want to hear. I am the bearer of bad news on a daily basis. A seemingly minor diagnosis in terms of treatment or prognosis might seem like the end of the world to those on the receiving end. Receiving a diagnosis of dementia isn't what I would recognize as a mild condition, but in the early stages the signs and symptoms are pretty minimal, and many people continue to live their lives in more or less the same fashion. Except they're a little more prepared, a little more insightful into what challenges might lie ahead, and perhaps even a little more aware of how important the present moment is, a time when they are still largely well, given the next moment might not bring with it quite as much wellbeing.

Thankfully, there are a number of treatments available for some of the dementia types. We'll discuss these in the next chapter.

5
Treatments

The treatment of dementia is more than just pills. In fact, I would argue that my role, as a doctor, in the treatment of dementia is less important than all the other healthcare professionals and carers, both formal and informal. Treatment of dementia is more than just taking a tablet. It's a whole person, a team effort. As a doctor, my role is pretty small. What I mean by this is that, whilst we as doctors play an important role in the diagnosis and treatment of dementia, it seems to me that the care of those with these conditions involves much more than what I do as a clinician. It involves an army of professionals, teams of unsung heroes in terms of family members, friends, and informal carers.

The first thing I'd like to talk about is medications. They probably aren't the mainstay of treatment, but they have a role and can help in terms of symptom control and disease progression, for a while at least. We'll talk about the treatments for all dementias mentioned above.

Medications

There are a few medications available aimed at the direct treatment of dementia, and a number of others often used in the treatment of related symptoms, such as behavioural problems, depression, anxiety and insomnia. This list, once again, is by no means exhaustive, but it should provide you with a good idea of what treatments you might expect to receive from your doctor. Most of them are licensed for Alzheimer's disease. You'll often be trialled on them by your specialist, after which your family doctor or general practitioner may take over the prescribing and monitoring of them.

Where possible I've used the generic names for the medications. Medications have a brand name which often varies between countries, and isn't always called the same thing. A drug should only have one generic name. This is the name of the chemical, for the want of a better term, the main active ingredient found in the tablet. The main medications involved in the treatment of dementia are: donepezil, rivastigmine, galantamine and memantine. Please bear in mind that the following is not a substitute for seeking medical attention, or getting advice from a trained medical professional or pharmacist.

Donepezil

Donepezil is a tablet used for the treatment of mild to moderate Alzheimer's disease. It works by stopping the breakdown of a neurotransmitter called acetylcholine, by an enzyme called acetylcholinesterase. Neurotransmitters are like cellular relay runners, or, perhaps more accurately, the baton. They are released from the ends of nerves, either to meet other nerves (called synapses) or they meet muscles (called neuromuscular junctions). Acetylcholine has a number of functions in the body. It's released from the neuromuscular junction and is important for voluntary movement. In the autonomic nervous system, the part of the nervous system we don't need to think about for it to get to work, it is involved in the fight or flight response. This is the response that keeps us safe from danger or perceived threat. In the central nervous system (basically our brain and spinal cord), it's involved in arousal, reward, alert, attention, learning, memory and sleep. A pretty important little chemical.

It's thought that by increasing the level of this chemical available in the brain (by preventing its breakdown), some of these areas mentioned above may not be quite so negatively impacted upon.

It's been shown that medications for Alzheimer's, such as donepezil, slow the progression of the condition. It's not a cure. It doesn't give back what's gone, but it might help us keep what's there for a little longer. We tend to keep people on the medication for as long as we think they'll derive benefit from it. In general, it helps improve the condition for up to about 18 months, but it's felt best to keep taking the medication while clear benefit is derived. We might only consider stopping it right towards the end of life.

As with all medications, there are side effects. At medical school I was once advised that, if I couldn't remember an answer when asked what side effects a drug might have, I was to respond 'nausea, vomiting, rash and death', which is probably true of every medication I've either taken myself or prescribed another. While it's important to read the little leaflet you get with a medication (I mean, I do it all the time), you'd probably never take any medication ever if you worried about all the potential side effects.

Donepezil tends to cause diarrhoea, nausea and headaches in some people. It can increase the risk of catching colds, apparently, reduce a person's appetite, cause hallucinations, agitation, aggression, collapse, dizziness, insomnia, vomiting, abdominal discomfort, rash, itching, muscle cramps, urinary incontinence, fatigue and pain. I told you there'd be a rash . . .

In most cases I meet, people don't really get side effects outside a slightly gippy tummy, but we do need to let people know big horrible things that are rare, and minor things that happen a lot. Like nausea, vomiting, rash, etc. When you get your first prescription, read the tiny leaflet with the impossibly small print and, if you have any concerns, have a chat with your doctor or friendly neighbourhood pharmacist.

Rivastigmine

Rivastigmine is another tablet that's generally referred to as an anticholinesterase, like donepezil. It comes in a tablet form, and also a patch. Which is handy for those who don't like taking tablets, or struggle to swallow them. Again it's been shown to help reduce the speed of deterioration and we'll keep prescribing it as long as there appears to be a benefit. In terms of side effects, reduced appetite, agitation, confusion, anxiety, dizziness, headaches, sleepiness and tremor, nausea, vomiting, diarrhoea, abdominal pain, indigestion, sweating, fatigue and weight loss are possible, and are either classed as common or very common. However, most people I meet seem to get on just fine. Being started on a medication isn't a one-way trip, and if you don't get on with it, it can be stopped. However, I would suggest you do this in discussion with your doctor, as some medications can make you feel unwell if you stop them abruptly. Given that symptoms of dementia tend to slide a little on stopping, it's always worth chatting it through with your doctor.

Galantamine

Galantamine is another medication used in the treatment of dementia, particularly mild to moderate dementia. It's also been shown to reduce the speed of deterioration for a period of time. It comes in both capsule and an oral solution, so again it can be useful for those with swallowing difficulties. As with the other medications mentioned above, there are a host of potential side effects, most of which I haven't seen in my patients. That said, someone's got to get them. As with the other medications, this list is by no means exhaustive and shouldn't be read instead of the patient information leaflet you get with your meds. Side effects include a reduced appetite, hallucinations, depression, collapse, dizziness, tremor, sleepiness and lethargy, slow movements, high blood pressure, abdominal discomfort, diarrhoea and indigestion.

Memantine

Memantine works in a slightly different way to the other medications, namely as a 'voltage dependent moderate-affinity uncompetitive NMDA receptor antagonist', which is a bit of a mouthful. Again licensed for use in Alzheimer's disease, it has a number of side effects. Namely drug hypersensitivity reactions (e.g. rash), sleepiness, dizziness, balance problems, high blood pressure, indigestion, constipation, a change in liver function tests, and headache. Once again, these are still reasonably rare, and if in doubt check with your doctor or pharmacist.

The medications we've just mentioned are used for the treatment of the main symptom of dementia, which is memory difficulties. They work to a point, keep our memory intact a little longer, and generally slow the progression of the condition, particularly with reference to Alzheimer's disease. We leave people on them as long as they appear to derive benefit, although in most cases the evidence is for about 18 months of benefit at most. This doesn't mean that the medications don't work longer, but just means we don't necessarily have the science to back it up. That said, with more and more people on the medication for longer than the trials, we should be able to generate enough experience with the medications to see if they have long term benefits.

The next group of medications are used to help with what are termed 'behavioural and psychological symptoms of dementia' (BPSD). This is a pretty general term that includes symptoms such as agitation, confusion, anger, irritability, depression, wandering and 'challenging' behaviour. Medications probably aren't the be all and end all of the treatment of such symptoms.

I don't get angry very often. I think perhaps three times in my life have I been really angry, and they were all to do with election results. But I digress. I suppose what I'm trying to say is there's a reason we might get angry. There's a reason I might not want to sit next to a particular person, or why I might want to get out of a chair, or why I might want to sit outside, have a cup of tea or scratch myself. All behaviour stems from a thought or a feeling, a response to some internal manifestation and awareness of our current state of being. What is really difficult is how to express how we feel if we can't communicate as well, or aren't certain how we feel.

Equally challenging is interpreting what a change in behaviour means given these communication challenges. There is a real challenge in resisting the impulse to medicate as a first resort, when really it might be a case of keeping an eye on things, watching and waiting, or looking for other things that might cause problems, such as physical illness. Infections can cause considerable confusion, pain can make us angry or agitated. Our physical and mental wellbeing are explicitly linked, in fact one could argue they're one and the same.

Sometimes, it might be something as simple as not wanting to sit in a particular location, or next to a particular person. Many residential care establishments have a lot of communal space. There are plenty of people I'd rather not spend time with, and I'm sure many would say the same of me, yet in such establishments people are thrust together, their only common feature being cognitive impairment. Realities diverging. Is it any wonder that people develop changes in behaviour that those of us in a caring profession can't comprehend?

There are a number of medications that we use for BPSDs (I'll use that for shorthand). For relief from simple pain we could include paracetamol. Cheap, cheerful, mostly safe and good for most mild pain. There's a solid body of evidence to suggest the use of paracetamol helps with agitation and behavioural problems in people with dementia. There's mixed evidence to support its use.

Infections can cause a marked change in behaviour, and the infections I tend to see most often are urinary or chest infections. These are usually treated with antibiotics but, even then, it's difficult to say if that is truly what's causing the behavioural changes.

The group of drugs we tend to use for BPSD are called antipsychotic drugs. I think treating these symptoms with medication engenders a feeling of guilt among some of us in the profession, particularly as we don't have a lot else to use. Past generations of doctors may have used sedatives, the 'chemical cosh' for want of a better term. Again, what else was there, and how do you know how to help someone who appears to be suffering, in anguish or despair, without truly knowing what's wrong? We now know that they are generally of little benefit, although occasionally low doses of benzodiazepines, such as lorazepam, can be used for the short-term alleviation of distress and other BPSD in urgent cases.

Antipsychotic medications are a group of drugs used in the treatment of psychosis, that is a change in the mental state causing confusion, delusions (believing things that aren't real), and hallucinations (sensing things that aren't really there). We have a tenuous grasp on reality at the best of times, and it doesn't take much for this to slip. All experience is essentially constructed in our brains, based on information that our senses convey. This information is probably only a fraction of what is truly out there, and our brains have to choose what we perceive, what we notice and attend to, and what we can put to one side.

The drug I tend to use in BPSD in dementia (but should be avoided in dementia with Lewy bodies as they make problems worse) is risperidone. It's meant to be used in short-term alleviation of BPSD but, in reality, some people stay on them a little longer. It's usually taken as a tablet, and given at regular intervals over the course of a day. Forms of it come in solution and an injection, but I've personally never used the long-acting injection for this patient group. The solution occasionally comes in handy for people with swallowing difficulties.

In terms of side effects, there are plenty. In no particular order, the more common ones include pneumonia, bronchitis, upper respiratory chest infections, sinusitis, urinary tract infections, influenza, ear infections, increased appetite (which is sometimes handy in people with poor dietary intakes), increased or decreased weight, reduced appetite (sometimes good in those with obesity), poor sleep, depression, sedation and increased sleepiness, Parkinsonism (hence the need to avoid in dementia with Lewy bodies), restlessness and agitation, tremor and movement disorders, blurred vision, conjunctivitis, fast heart rate, shortness of breath, nasal congestion, abdominal pain, nausea, vomiting, constipation, indigestion, dry mouth, toothache, cough, nose bleeds, rashes, muscle spasm and urinary incontinence. And these are just those classed as 'common'. As as result of these side effects, limited benefit and potential harms, we try and avoid the use of antipsychotic medication if at all possible. You can see why we would prefer people to only remain on them for the shortest time possible. That's much the same for all medication. We only really want to prescribe them for as long as is clinically needed, in the lowest effective dose required to provide symptomatic relief or have a meaningful impact on the disease in question.

Other antipsychotic medication used in the treatment of BPSDs include aripiprazole, olanzapine, quetiapine and, potentially, clozapine. These are all drugs that might have some impact on the behaviour of someone suffering from troubling behavioural and psychological symptoms of dementia, although I tend not to use them very often. Our prescribing decisions are, in part, due to familiarity, as well as safety and efficacy. I avoid clozapine as it requires regular blood tests to monitor for potential side effects affecting the blood, and this is probably not of great benefit in people with advancing dementia. Having a blood test isn't always a lot of fun, and if you're not aware of the reasoning behind it, it does seem a little unnecessary. I tend to find it is used more often in people with severe psychosis, rather than dementia.

The one drug that has been used in the UK for the treatment of BPSDs is quetiapine, which we try to avoid if possible. It became rather popular for some time among the medical fraternity, and I'm not entirely certain why. It can be sedating which is sometimes useful, especially when given at night, and it can help with treatment of anxiety and psychosis, but it isn't really any use in the treatment of BPSDs and can cause side effects. These include anaemia (which is a low haemoglobin), a reduced white cell count (which is part of the blood system that fights infection), abnormal thyroid function (a gland in the neck that helps control metabolism), cholesterol changes, blood glucose problems, nightmares, suicidal thoughts and behaviour, dizziness, movement disorders, speech problems, palpitations and a fast heart rate, low blood pressure, shortness of breath, dry mouth, constipation, sore throat, swelling, fever, chest pain, tiredness, increased falls, abnormal liver function tests, swelling, irritability, and fever. Other side effects are possible and, once again, this list is not exhaustive. Not everyone will get a drug side effect, and especially not all of them simultaneously. If we got every medication side effect, we'd probably rather stay ill.

Despite these potential side effects, quetiapine still serves a purpose, and we tend to use it at very low doses. I use quetiapine as an adjunct in depression as it often helps people sleep when given at night, and when given at low doses it is easily tolerated and tends to be easy enough to stop.

Depression and anxiety are not uncommon in dementia and neuro-degenerative conditions in general. Sometimes early dementia and depression can be confused. We might diagnose someone with dementia, simply on the grounds of age and symptoms, when what they really are is depressed. Some may be diagnosed with depression, particularly if their cognition is relatively spared, but what they have is the early stages of dementia. Depression is a very common problem, irrespective of underlying dementia or otherwise, for a variety of reasons. In the context of any of the diseases considered in this book, it's not just being ill that makes us depressed. We are what we think, and our thoughts originate in the myriad of synapses and neurons that fill our brain. We are the culmination of millions of chemical processes, each thought and feeling originating in chemistry and electricity. If those neurons, chemicals and signals aren't working well, then neither do we. Depression is another illness, caused by a derangement of fault in our chemistry, so is it any surprise that we become depressed? It's not just about feeling sad because we are unwell.

Depression, much like dementia, isn't just treated with medications. Psychological therapies play an important role, but medications are also useful. There are a number of different classes of antidepressant medication, the most common class I tend to use in all patient groups is the SSRI, or selective serotonin reuptake inhibitor. The first of its class was fluoxetine, and for the past couple of decades or so they've been a pillar of treatment for depressive symptoms. They work by increasing the amount of serotonin available in the brain, the lack of which is thought to contribute to depression. They are usually taken once a day, and can be given with other classes of antidepressants. Examples include citalopram, sertraline, fluoxetine and escitalopram. As with the other classes of drug thus far mentioned, there's potential for many side effects. The commonest ones I tend to see with the SSRIs are nausea, bowel disturbance, and worsening anxiety in the first few weeks, but these generally settle. SSRIs come in tablet form, some in liquid drops, and some in tablets that melt in the mouth. Doses vary between medications, so don't get too hung up on whether 5mg of escitalopram is less than 50mg sertraline. It's like comparing apples and oranges. I get a lot of patients who seem to think that because the number is lower, they're somehow having a milder dose of antidepressant. It doesn't work that way.

There are other medications that may be of use in treating the behavioural and psychological symptoms of dementia, in terms of treating depression in particular. A drug that's commonly used, either as a sole antidepressant or in addition to SSRIs, is mirtazapine. Mirtazapine works by increasing noradrenaline and serotonin to be available in the synapses, the gaps between nerve cells. Rather than preventing the uptake of these neurotransmitters, this medication increases their concentration, which is thought to help in terms of treating depression. Naturally there are many potential side effects, but the most commonly noticed ones are increased appetite and increasing sleepiness. Consequently, it's a really useful adjunct in people who might have poor sleep, poor appetite *and* depression. These aren't uncommon in the context of dementia. I recall the first time I prescribed mirtazapine. I know I should remember more interesting things, such as my children's birthdays, or literally anything my wife tells me, but I remember this occasion. I was a junior doctor on the ward. We had a patient admitted with a medical problem, probably an infection of some form. We started her on mirtazapine and, as her admission was a few weeks, we had the opportunity to see the impact. It was noted that her appetite and sleep were markedly improved, even if she didn't feel much different, at least initially.

I also tend to use mirtazapine alongside SSRI antidepressants as an adjunct to help with sleep and appetite, if I feel that these symptoms are also a potential problem in addition to depressive symptoms. For many, an SSRI-plus-mirtazapine combination works well in terms of mood, sleep and appetite.

We've talked about the key medications for the treatment of Alzheimer's disease, we've talked about what medications might be used for the behavioural and psychological symptoms of dementia, and what might be useful in the treatment of depression. While medications undoubtedly play a role in the treatment of dementia, they aren't the be all and end all. If I can treat a condition with lifestyle or behavioural changes, I'd much rather do that than use a medication. Chapter 7 discusses how we help people without medication.

6
Behavioural and psychological symptoms of dementia

Behavioural or psychological symptoms of dementia affect most people with dementia at some point, and they can cause considerable distress in caregivers and patients alike. People can become restless, agitated, repetitive, wander off, lose interest in things, or even spend time screaming. I recall many a time when I'd walk onto a ward to find acutely unwell people with dementia manifesting many of these behaviours. It's distressing for all concerned, and as a very junior doctor I had a deep desire to help, but no real way of actually making a difference.

Given that dementia, in general, is a progressive condition, BPSDs tend to worsen with time, requiring greater support both in terms of healthcare and social needs, increasing the cost of care, and increasing carer stress. Looking after someone with advancing dementia is intensely difficult, there's no let-up, and it causes a lot of problems with carers' health.

BPSDs are often associated with a rapid reduction in cognition, such as you might see after a fresh vascular event in vascular dementia. They get worse as the illness progresses, meaning the person affected will need more help with their everyday activities, ultimately leading to an increasing need for care and even residential care in many cases. We tend to see increasing hospital admissions with advancing dementia, looking after many of the associated problems that occur when our brains don't work as well. In general, quality of life suffers, for the patient and their loved ones. This is not an easy thing to experience.

Aside from medications, there are a number of other approaches that can help reduce the burden of the disease on those directly affected and those providing a caring role.

Non-drug options should, ideally, be the first-line treatment. Medications play a role, but it's short-lived, not immediately noticeable, and ultimately causes side effects. Non-drug options have fewer side effects, and are usually much safer than medications.

Therapy options such as music therapy, aromatherapy, exercise, individually tailored activities, reality orientation, art therapy, behavioural therapies and a host of other options can all help, to some degree, to reduce the impact that the symptoms of dementia have on those suffering from the condition and those in a caring role.

7
Non-pharmacological treatments

There are a number of treatment options available to try to minimize the use of medication in the treatment of dementia. While most people with a common cause of dementia, such as Alzheimer's, are likely to be on some form of medication, there are a number of options available to help alleviate the potential burden that the disease brings, especially in terms of behavioural and psychological symptoms of dementia.

For a long time, I used to get the impression that non-drug treatment of dementia, particularly in the context of residential care or nursing homes, was to invite assorted retired cruise ship singers to sing wartime hits. If or when I'm in a similar establishment, if they start singing wartime melodies, I shall be most disgruntled; I want mid-eighties onwards. And why is there always a daytime TV show on about how to renovate a house/sell a house/buy a house in the UK/somewhere hot? Almost everything on daytime television in a nursing home seems to be about house renovations. If you want to learn how to make a profit from property, spend some time sitting in a residential home.

I'm being flippant. Modern dementia care is evolving, away from simply corralling people into the same space, irrespective of what people liked to do or who they liked to spend their time with in their 'premorbid' condition. It's now much more person-centred, and the approach to non-drug treatment is a little more sophisticated than daytime property shows and the hits of Vera Lynn.

In terms of non-drug options, there are three broad areas of concern: the behavioural and psychological symptoms of dementia, signs of distress and how to facilitate communication.

As a doctor, our first step is to detect what might be causing the change in symptoms, such as pain, agitation, constipation, infection, or medication side effects. We've mentioned how simple infections can cause problems in terms of confusion.

There are lots of different causes of confusion and we can find out many relatively simply.

We should consider the surroundings of the person exhibiting the change in behaviour. Is it simply a reaction to the environment, for example temperature, lighting, background noise, etc.? Simple environmental changes might be all that is needed to alleviate the suffering of the individual concerned.

It might be that the change in behaviour might be related to a specific event or episode. I've met a number of people who became agitated when their loved ones visited. This causes consternation for the loved one as well as those in a caring role. People might respond negatively to personal care. Imagine how you might respond if, for some unknown reason, someone appeared in your room to give you a flannel wash. I'd be somewhat surprised, to say the least.

In terms of behavioural and psychological symptoms, they tend to lessen if people remain active, engaged, and involved in an activity that matches their premorbid interests. 'Premorbid' is a strange term, but it basically refers to a time before a disease kicked in; A time before the disease became apparent. Changes in behaviour could be due to the disease process itself; changes in the brain, particularly affecting the frontal lobes, can cause changes in our ability to tone our behaviour down. We might notice changes in behaviour due to care given, surroundings, and how people spend their time, not just physical health problems. When you think about it, it's not too surprising, is it? Our behaviours are influenced by a variety of internal cues. Thoughts and feelings trigger behaviours. So hunger, thirst, feeling hot or cold, pain and so on will influence our demeanour. Emotional states such as sadness, happiness and anger all have a direct effect on our actions.

This is all well and good when we can communicate the state of our inner environment to others directly, usually through speech, but if this is impaired it's up to those around us to hazard the best guess. It's not easy but, over time, it might become more apparent.

Spending time with our loved ones may help. For some, social interaction is sufficient to help moderate the impact of behavioural and psychological symptoms. Communicating, even if it's a cup of tea and a chat, is a simple way for all of us to feel connected and valued. Over time we can pick up subtle, or some not so subtle, non-verbal cues that the person we're sitting with may not be entirely happy or content, or help us identify their needs a little more easily.

There are a number of approaches, and many of us might use them without being overtly aware. Some might involve more active input or engagement from either the carer or the patient. It must be said that there's variable evidence for many of the therapies and strategies mentioned in the following section.

Some people try memory training activities, others engage in mental or social stimulation (which is called life, isn't it?) and physical exercise. Whether it does much to change the outcome is hard to prove, but given that doing things to keep us stimulated, spending time with people we like, doing things we enjoy, and getting a bit of fresh air and exercise makes many of us feel good, perhaps we should try it irrespective of what the scientific evidence suggests.

Medicine loves a bit of evidence, but it's very hard to get objective, 'gold-standard evidence' in a lot of non-drug approaches to dementia care. The key type of study that tends to give the highest quality of evidence is the 'randomized-controlled trial'. Basically, this involves comparing an intervention or therapy to another therapy or none at all, and is usually 'blinded', which means neither the participant nor the investigator know what the intervention is. That way, you can reduce the risk of bias creeping into the data. It's really hard to not know that you're doing a brain training exercise, listening to music or carrying out exercise, so it's hard to generate enough good quality data to say that a particular intervention has benefits for dementia treatment. Also, studies usually show how a particular intervention affects the population studied, but how that affects an individual is harder to predict.

Say a study shows that dance helps reduce agitation in people with dementia. Now, it might be possible to show that many people in a group benefit from a little bit of time doing the tango or the American smooth, but it would personally drive me mad.

Whether that would change after a diagnosis of dementia, who knows, but I can't imagine that being the case. Take me for a walk in my favourite place on the edge of the Cambridgeshire Fens and this would work for me, but I'm aware this isn't for everyone. In no particular order, once again, here are some of the therapies that have been shown to work. The vast majority of these interventions are aimed at causing improvements in the behavioural and psychological symptoms of dementia.

The aim of treatment of dementia, be it the core symptoms of memory failure or the wider symptoms of behavioural and psychological symptoms, is to improve or maintain quality of life for both the person affected and their wider family; to retain the ability to continue carrying out their everyday activities, as far as is possible; and to address any additional changes that have been noted. This includes treating depression, anxiety, sleep disturbance, agitation, aggression, etc.

There are a number of more structured approaches that have been tried. The first up for consideration is something called **reality orientation**. The aim of this is to work with the affected person to ensure they are aware, as much as is possible, of lots of features we take for granted as real. This includes group sessions reminding people of time, place, and general features of reality. It may help improve some cognitive and behavioural elements of the disease.

Cognitive stimulation therapy is pretty much what it says on the tin: therapy aimed at stimulating a person's cognition. It might include word games and puzzles, and in general it seems to help improve cognition to some degree, improve quality of life and lead to an improved general sense of wellbeing. It's also been shown to improve planning and recall, and reduce the frequency and severity of behavioural problems. It tends to be used in those with mild to moderate dementia, as those with more advanced disease may find it difficult to engage with the process.

There are a number of psychological therapies out there that might help people with dementia. It's generally difficult to carry out studies in the area, as mentioned previously, so the evidence base for these therapies isn't always as robust as we'd like it to be. Medicine has traditionally been a profession lacking in evidence, at least in the scientific sense, but modern medicine relies on collecting data to show that a particular medication, therapy or operation is of benefit. If there's no decent data, a treatment is hard to recommend until such time that we have evidence either for or against a particular intervention.

Reminiscence therapy involves spending time recalling the past, using aids such as photography, familiar items, music or memories. In many forms of dementia, recent events are often hard to remember. Short-term memory is often significantly impaired, whereas long held memories are easily accessible. Reminiscence therapy has been shown to help improve mood, but it's effects on cognitive function are less certain. There might be a small short-term improvement, and it might help alleviate some of the symptoms of depression to a mild degree. The aim of this type of therapy is to use past experience to help people in the present. I don't know about you, but there are some experiences I'd rather not relive. Times when I've been hurt, times when I've hurt others. Times of sorrow, anger and despair. We've all had these. Even times of happiness can often be tinged with sadness. Recalling loved ones who are no longer with us can feel somewhat bitter-sweet. Nostalgia means 'pain for the past' and, from a personal point of view, I prefer to live in the present. Yet, for those of us whose present is painful, patchy or just downright confusing, perhaps reminiscence therapy is useful. The aim is to use positive, personally significant memories. Perhaps I am being a little disingenuous. The past might be littered with hurt or pain, but it can also be filled with joy and pleasure. We just have to be picky about the past that we entertain.

If it were me undergoing reminiscence therapy, it would be the time I met my wife. She was the most beautiful person I ever saw and, despite never needing to visit the ward on which she was working, I'd still find some excuse to go and see her. I might have needed to look after a patient on her ward once or twice. Eventually, after several weeks of trying to find a reason to see her, I asked her out. I'm not sure HR would have liked me basically trying to get a date while on work time, particularly as I was one of the few junior doctors covering the wards that weekend.

Perhaps I'd think about the birth of my children, both of whom I love with all my heart. Perhaps it might be all the great times I've spent with my friends, my family, the summers spent with my late grandmother, or maybe that holiday in Ibiza when I lost my Han Solo figure in the sand on the beach. See, not all memories are joyous.

Reminiscence therapy isn't just about passive recall. It might involve art, music or artefacts of importance to provide mental stimulation. As with many of these therapies, it's hard to prove that they are of benefit, but reminiscence therapy is thought to help improve pleasure, cause a degree of cognitive stimulation, and increase general levels of wellbeing.

Validation therapy involves providing validation for a person's behaviours, rather than challenging. In this therapy, it's thought that many of the episodes of confusion or agitation are due to stress, boredom, loneliness and a desire to escape reality. The aim is to validate, or essentially agree with what the patient feels and the behaviours displayed. Sort of 'going along with it' rather than constantly reinforcing what may be the genuine reality to the one experienced by the person with dementia. It's thought that it helps alleviate stress, promotes a degree of contentment and reduces behavioural disturbance, at least to a mild degree. It's less interested in facts, and more interested in feelings. Validation therapy is less reliant on accuracy and truth, in terms of orientation in time and place, instead it emphasizes empathy with possible meanings within potentially confused communication. Emotion trumps fact in this case, but it's hard to prove that this is useful in terms of scientific studies. It does seem to reduce negative moods, improve behaviour and contentment, but it's not certain as to the long-term benefit. It might also miss actual needs. Are the behaviour changes missing out on genuine, physical needs such as pain, thirst, hunger or a need for mental stimulation?

Reality orientation helps people remember facts about themselves and their environment, and can be done either individually or in groups. It could involve constant reorientation, such as signposts and notices and other aide memoires, or intermittent correction and orientation. The benefits are uncertain. It might help people appear orientated, but it could also remind the person affected with dementia that they're ill, or have lost a degree of independence, or are in a nursing or residential home.

There are some suggestions that it can, initially, cause a drop in mood. Carers might become frustrated with repeated attempts to re-orientate those they look after. I've seen numerous examples of increased agitation brought about by a well-meaning loved one, usually talking very loudly and slowly to someone with dementia, saying 'you're at the doctor's...the doctor's'. In terms of the long-term effect, it's hard to say. Given the deterioration that is inevitable with dementia, I'm not certain this helps people stay oriented in the long term.

Reality orientation aims to reduce confusion and behavioural symptoms by repeatedly orientating people in time and place. It may be done informally, with care staff or family members reminding a person of time, place etc., or in groups in a more formal setting with games, calendars, discussions etc. It has some effect on cognition and behaviour, but to a mild extent.

Occupational therapy, therapy aimed at promoting independence and adapting to changing abilities, has been shown to reduce aggression, agitation and depression, and improve quality of life. We all change, and our abilities change as we progress through life. As we get older, irrespective of disease or diagnosis, we find it more of a challenge to do things we used to take for granted. Occupational therapy provides assistance and strategies with carrying out everyday activities, such as washing or dressing, or adaptations to make our house safer and more amenable to our needs as our abilities change. Technological adaptations such as phones with large buttons, speed dials for relatives, even phones with pictures of loved ones on can help people remain independent and in their own home for longer. Strategies to help with meal planning, adaptations to the building (such as easier access steps, grab rails, wet rooms, toilet seat rises or even raised toilets), aide memoires, and care alarms can all help build a world around us that allows us to operate despite our changing abilities. Increasingly, cameras can be used in the home to ensure the safety of our loved ones. It might seem like an invasion of privacy, and perhaps it is, but changing and improving technology can help us remain independent for longer.

We have a camera at our front door. It's really handy when a parcel is being delivered, or if I'm in the garden and can't hear the doorbell. A lot of the time it shows cats passing in front of it in the middle of the night. I never knew my driveway was a hotbed of feline nocturnal activity, but there you go. It even went off when a bee buzzed around it. Perhaps this isn't that useful for you, but if you have a loved one who is prone to wandering out, or you're worried about who might be coming to see them, then technology such as this can be very helpful. The newer generation cameras even have two-way sound, so you can talk to people who appear on camera. Whether this is a good or bad thing in the context of dementia remains to be seen.

Tailored activity programmes are just that. Activities tailored to a person's needs and things they find enjoyable. It should probably be called 'doing stuff you like', but a 'tailored activity programme' does sound a bit more formal, and probably is to some extent. An activity is selected based on a person's abilities, interests and perhaps past roles, simplified if necessary, and adapted as these abilities change. In general terms, it's been shown to reduce the behavioural and psychological symptoms of dementia. It's probably not much of a surprise. I think we're all generally happier doing stuff we enjoy. I'm a much nicer person after a walk in the Fens with the dog, or a bit of meditation. And much more grumpy after a day of meetings. Just because someone has dementia, doesn't mean that their capacity for enjoyment diminishes.

Music therapy has been shown to reduce agitation. Be it live, pre-recorded, or interactive, people like music. Group music therapy has been shown to reduce anxiety and agitation, particularly in moderate to severe dementia. There are similar therapies available. Art therapy, for instance, aims to provide potentially meaningful multisensory stimulation, and may well help increase social interaction when performed in a group setting. It provides the opportunity for self-expression, and such chances may become less prevalent as dementia progresses. Whether it makes a difference, who knows, but if it brings someone pleasure, I would suggest they keep doing it.

Music therapy involves engaging in musical activities, be it individually or in groups. It may involve actively creating music, or simply listening to it. It's been shown to increase wellbeing, social interactions, autobiographical memory (remembering the song in relation to past life experiences), reduced behavioural problems, and reduced agitation (providing the music chosen is individualized to taste).

Psychological therapies, such as Cognitive behavioural therapy (CBT), might be helpful to those with dementia in the early stages, as might interpersonal therapy. CBT ultimately allows us to look at how our thoughts, feelings and behaviours are all linked, and Interpersonal therapy (IPT) looks at how relationships between ourselves and others can affect our mental state. To some extent, we need to be able to think to a fair degree to get the best out of these therapies, but as dementia progresses this might be more of a struggle.

Activity therapy, such as sport, drama or dance, has been shown to provide health benefits in terms of physical fitness, reducing falls, and improving mood, confidence, mental health and sleep. This makes sense. There aren't many people I would recommend not to exercise. It's been shown to be of benefit in pretty much any medical condition you can think of (within reason), even when we thought it might not be a great idea to be too active in the past. Exercise is good for us. Plus, exercising in the daytime has been shown to reduce daytime agitation and night time restlessness in people with dementia.

Behavioural therapy relies upon identifying and learning what behaviours are triggered by what stimuli, and adopting strategies to reduce or eliminate that behaviour. After a period of assessment, triggers and reinforcements of potentially distressing behaviour are identified and made clear to the patient, and this is usually charted by a therapist of some form. Interventions, ways and means of preventing or minimizing the impact of this behaviour are implemented depending on these findings. The aim is to take account of the patient's preferences, the context of the behaviour and how to reinforce more potentially positive behaviours. It has been shown to reduce wandering and incontinence, and particular behaviours typical to that person.

I've seen the impact of this sort of approach in residential placements, but on a more informal level. I've certainly never seen a therapist in a residential home, not from a psychological point of view. Care home staff, particularly experienced ones, are usually very able to identify the stimuli for potentially adverse, negative or challenging behaviours. I've seen plenty of examples where experienced staff have been able to identify and prevent behaviours becoming problematic. In one home I used to visit, I would see a lady repeatedly folding towels. It was a part of her former job; I think she might have been a member of the housekeeping staff in a hotel. So the staff would provide her with a trolley and towels, and away she would go. They'd noticed that she'd repeatedly fold napkins at lunch, and if there was something that wasn't folded, she'd give it a go, whether the person near her wanted it folded or not. Her dementia was at least moderate and, while her ability to communicate verbally had declined, she was mobile and able to express her needs in other ways. One of those needs was folding. Staff noticed her agitation, intervened and provided a simple task that she could do uninterrupted, without affecting others in a negative fashion. It didn't require anything more than staff being vigilant and having access to clean laundry. And this didn't involve a medication to help her feel calm or at peace. As far as I know, there are no significant side effects from folding towels.

Another example of this, perhaps also on a more informal level, also occurred in the context of a residential home. People are often put together with people they may not normally associate with. They might be forced to engage with activities that they would rather avoid. I would frequently see people become less agitated if they moved location. A simple move that changed behaviour, that didn't require a medication or specialist knowledge. It just needed the care staff to notice.

Similar approaches can quite easily occur in the home context, particularly when being looked after by loved ones. When people we care for, people we love develop dementia, they become a different version of themselves. This is hard for many of us to accept, but none of us are permanent. We're just passing through, and even who we think of as ourselves changes over time. We are none of us the same person as when we were born. Life etches itself upon us, physically and mentally, and the same can be said for disease. Any disease, accident or illness can have the potential to change us, and dementia is no exception. Over time, living with someone with dementia, we begin to notice the new them. The changes may be subtle and, over time, awareness develops of what triggers and cues may lead to what novel behaviours.

Complementary Therapies

Other therapies might well help people with dementia, at least in terms of underlying behaviour and psychological symptoms. Aromatherapy may help with some of the difficult behaviours. Lavender and melissa balsam have been looked at in research. They seem to help reduce agitation to some degree and, given that they are largely free of side effects when inhaled, seem to provide a useful adjunct or alternative to pharmacological therapy in some cases.

Bright light therapy, basically where something akin to a SADS lamp is used, can help reduce the fluctuation in diurnal rhythm that some with dementia undergo. Essentially, some people with dementia become more agitated or active towards the end of the day, often referred to as 'sundowning'. I'm not really sure why this happens, but it does, and it isn't particularly uncommon.

Multi-sensory therapy uses a room designed to provide sensory stimulation. You might have seen or heard of these rooms. The sort of thing that you might have seen in special schools or even soft-play areas, containing lights and fibre optic cables, as well as textured materials, sounds and even smells. I must admit I've not seen this in any particular residential placements I've visited, and I wonder if there's all that much evidence for it in this patient group.

The National Institute of Health and Care Excellence (NICE) has guidelines on the diagnosis and care of people with dementia. The guidelines advise on the use of cognitive stimulation therapy, group reminiscence therapy and occupational therapy for mild to moderate dementia. They advise against acupuncture, ginkgo biloba, vitamin E, cognitive training, interpersonal therapy or non-invasive brain stimulation.

In terms of complementary or alternative treatments, aroma-therapy, which involves the use of scented oils, has been shown to a limited degree to help with agitation and behavioural symptoms.

So, in summary, what options are there for helping people with dementia cope with the symptoms of dementia, particularly the behavioural and psychological symptoms? In my experience, it seems that a mixed bag of strategies is applied to help reduce the impact of dementia in general. I often see care staff apply a mixture of approaches when trying to ameliorate the impact of this set of conditions, be it orientating people to reality, helping them reminisce, keeping an eye out for things that might cause behaviour to change, and adapting the environment to fit a changing inner reality. The treatment of dementia isn't really about a tablet or a pill, there's no surgery that will cure this disease, it's about changing the environment around them. The next few chapters help us discover what practical steps can be taken to help smooth out the path that we follow when diagnosed with dementia.

8
Power of attorney

To paraphrase one of my favourite fictional doctors (Leonard McCoy from Star Trek), 'I'm a doctor, not a lawyer', but I'll do my best to talk about the principles of something called power of attorney.

When we are well, we are pretty much expected to be able to manage our own affairs and make our own decisions. We are expected to be able to get done the sorts of things we all take for granted, make our views known, put our opinions across. Dementia, over time, tends to rob us of these abilities. Our sense of independence, and our ability to voice that slowly ebbs away. Like the tide slowly heading out.

When we are young, and if we are fortunate, we have people there to look after us. Parents that love us, teachers to guide us, and others in a position of responsibility that we look up to. As we go through life we become those people, we are the teachers, the parents, the carers, but at the other end of life, who is there for us?

The role of the attorney is to provide a legally appointed person, or people, to help us manage our affairs or carry out actions on our behalf if we are no longer in a position to be able to do it for ourselves. The processes vary depending on where in the UK you are and, if overseas, I'm afraid I'm not much use to you.

Power of attorney, either called Enduring (this is an older system and, if I'm not mistaken, the system used in Northern Ireland) or Lasting power of attorney, allows us to represent people on their behalf to make decisions for them. It's a really useful legal framework, because it means we can get stuff done with the help of someone we trust.

In general terms, attorneys are appointed to allow people to make decisions about finances and property, or health and welfare. Have you ever tried to get someone else to act on your behalf on the phone to a bank? It's often a no go for obvious reasons. Having a power of attorney means you can get someone to act for you. There are a few technicalities, in some cases they need to be registered, and it's worth letting people you deal with know that a power of attorney exists.

As a doctor, it's really helpful to know that someone has this, as we will usually involve them in discussions regarding health and welfare. We commonly encountered this when discussing resuscitation. When I was growing up, there used to be a TV programme about a group of lifeguards that worked on a beach. You know the one. People would run in slow motion to rescue people on a beach. Usually someone playing volleyball, or messing about on a jet ski would get into a spot of bother, and somehow be unconscious and need resuscitation. One of the aforementioned lifeguards would bounce up and down on someone's chest, breathe into their face and, as if by magic, they'd awaken unharmed and be able to dash off to return to whatever apparently risk laden activity they were engaging in. No need for hospital, no after care, no counselling, no spells in intensive care. Up they leapt and back to daily life, possibly bumping into David Hasselhoff in the process.

Anyway, cardiopulmonary resuscitation (CPR) isn't like that. For a start, you pretty much need a defibrillator to stand any chance of success, and I don't remember seeing any in that TV show. I'm not sure water and electricity mix too well. Also, you need to be able to reverse or somehow remove whatever it is that causes a person to need resuscitation, and in my experience that doesn't usually involve a jet ski. Or volleyball.

Resuscitation is pretty brutal, does not work most of the time, and should be viewed as a medical treatment like any other. It's amazing that it does work, but what is often required afterwards is a spell in hospital and a period of rehabilitation. We don't quite know what sort of condition a person will be in after a resuscitation effort.

Discussing CPR and end-of-life care is really difficult, but very important. We are none of us permanent, we're just passing through, and it's important for us to have a say in our departure, as much as we can. If we are unable to voice our wishes at that present moment, a power of attorney (for health and welfare) will be able to do that for us.

How we go about it varies upon where we are. You can often download the forms from the government website. Many people I meet have theirs arranged for them with a solicitor and, in some cases, the attorney is also a solicitor. We see that occasionally for finances and property, particularly if the person in question doesn't have any family members or other people they can trust.

Who you appoint as an attorney is down to you. In my experience it's usually a family member, or someone close to you that you trust. You often will need a back up attorney, called a replacement in the paperwork used in England. You might appoint more than one attorney. Once you've selected an attorney, there's usually a lot of paperwork, a visit to the solicitor, some more paperwork and a few bills. But having a power of attorney can make things an awful lot easier when it comes to dealing with our affairs, or having someone else help us.

One of the key features to be aware of is that these aren't permanent. You can change your mind or appoint another attorney, and it's only enacted once you're no longer in a position to make the particular decisions to which it pertains. When you're no longer able to make decisions is a tricky point to decide. If there's concern about our decision making, we tend to need our ability to make decisions assessed. This is called an assessment of capacity, and is often carried out with a professional familiar with such assessments. In essence, it's a process which someone, such as a doctor, social worker, specialist nurse, etc., carries out in order to check understanding and recall of a particular area of concern. If a person is deemed to lack capacity regarding a particular question, then it may be the attorney who is called upon to provide an answer.

The exact nature of the process involved varies a little between England and Wales, Scotland and Northern Ireland, and I'm not overly familiar with whatever equivalent processes there are in the rest of the world.

The process in England and Wales is the one I'm more familiar with. Essentially, you appoint one person (the attorney) to make decisions on your behalf. They ultimately control what happens if you have an accident or illness that means you can't decide for yourself.

The process is relatively straightforward. You fill in a form, appoint someone as an attorney, register your lasting power of attorney with something called the 'Office of the Public Guardian'. You can cancel it if it's no longer required.

Lasting power of attorney for health and welfare involves making decisions regarding washing, dressing and eating, as well as medical care (that's where I come in). It might also involve deciding whether to move into a care home, or even consider whether or not to remove life-sustaining treatment. They're only enacted when we are no longer able to make these decisions ourselves. Let's not forget that, just because we have an attorney, it doesn't mean the decision they're going to have to make is an easy one. These are some of the most difficult decisions we have to make for ourselves, never mind asking someone we trust or love to make them on our behalf. It isn't easy, and I would strongly recommend anyone making this decision for someone to talk it through.

Lasting power of attorney for property and financial affairs involves a lot of routine domestic financial management. It might involve managing bank accounts, bills, benefits and even selling your home. Once again, these aren't always easy decisions to make. Selling the family home, the bricks and mortar you've worked your whole life for, or have had handed down by previous generations, is not remotely easy.

Attorneys can be anyone over the age of 18 years, and may be a relative, friend, professional (e.g. solicitor), or spouse. Your attorney needs to have the mental capacity to make this decision, but at least in terms of England and Wales, doesn't necessarily need to reside within the UK or be a British citizen. That said, I've never seen an attorney appointed that doesn't currently live in the UK, merely for practical purposes. It's difficult, although not impossible, to manage the affairs of someone from across the oceans.

There are some important things to consider. Firstly, just how good do you think the person will be at managing your affairs or making decisions on your behalf? You might have a friend who is an awesome drinking buddy, or great fun to go and watch a game of football with, but who runs their life like an absolute car wreck. Personally, I'd go for the super-organized relative (but that's my personal view - I'd probably choose my wife, or my brother-in-law). You probably want to pick someone you know well, not the person you met last week at your flower arranging class. Do you trust them? Trust is a hard thing to gauge. I am generally very trusting but a terrible judge of character. You also need to consider just how happy are you for them to make decisions for you. If you think they've made some dubious decisions in the past, you probably don't want to be asking them to be your attorney.

You need one or more, they need to make decisions either independently or jointly, and a back-up (replacement) attorney is really useful. Making a lasting power of attorney can be done online or with a solicitor, and needs to have an attorney (or two), witnesses and someone called a 'certificate provider'. Basically, the certificate provider is someone who checks that you understand the whys and wherefores of the power of attorney and that you're not under any duress. Witnesses need to be over 18 years of age and need to be someone other than your attorney, which makes sense. In England and Wales, once completed, the power of attorney needs to be registered with the Office of the Public Guardian, either online or via post and, at the time of writing, it costs £82.00 to register. You'll find that solicitors tend to cost more than this, partly because of the preparatory work involved in drawing up a power of attorney. If you ask for a professional to be a certificate provider, this usually entails a further cost. The analogy I use is a bit like a tax return. You can do one yourself relatively inexpensively, but sometimes it's handy to have an accountant do one for you. Having someone aware of the ins and outs of the process is sometimes very useful.

9
Driving and dementia

One area that often causes concern in people, particularly when diagnosed with dementia, is driving. People immediately think that they will need to stop driving. While we've established that many types of dementia are progressive, this doesn't necessarily mean that all life must stop or radically alter at the time of diagnosis, particularly if diagnosed early on in the condition.

Driving is probably one of the riskiest things we do every day, particularly without thinking. We think nothing of jumping in our car, but driving is a physically and mentally complex task. We need to focus our attention, concentrate, have visuospatial awareness, solve problems, make judgements and decisions, and react and process information rapidly. But, once we can do it, we do many of these things almost unconsciously.

Today, I drove to memory clinic. I got into my car, put on my seat belt, depressed the clutch, started the engine, selected reverse gear, looked behind myself, checked for traffic on the street where I live, reversed out looking in my mirrors, selected first gear, surveyed my surroundings once again, checked my rear view mirror and set off forward. This is the first thirty seconds of my journey, and it relied upon all of those skills listed above.

As many forms of dementia progress, these skills become more and more difficult.

If you're diagnosed with dementia (and live in the UK), you need to notify the Driver and Vehicle Licensing Authority (DVLA). As a GP, the guidance we follow for fitness to drive is set out by the DVLA. They are the ultimate arbiter of whether we are permitted to drive on the UK's roads.

At the milder spectrum, or mild cognitive impairment (MCI), we tend not to see much driving impairment, and therefore there's no need to notify the DVLA. Let's not forget, MCI is cognitive impairment that tends not to cause too much in the way of impact on activities of daily living. Sometimes it is difficult to tell if there's any driving impairment. One common question I get asked in clinic is, 'am I safe to drive?'. It's pretty hard to answer sat in front of a computer, and I readily admit to not being the world's best driver. The DVLA guidance is useful in terms of when to stop driving in the context of a medical condition. It might be possible to surmise that someone is unable to drive due to a number of factors. This might be disorientation. If they get lost walking to the clinic, they probably shouldn't be driving about. Big, fast moving lumps of metal cause a lot more damage when not operated properly. Poor short-term memory, a lack of insight or impaired judgement might also call into question a person's ability to drive.

A clear diagnosis of dementia may also mean it's time to stop driving. The DVLA must be notified, but again it's hard to confirm if driving should stop. As per MCI, poor short term-memory, a lack of insight, poor judgement and disorientation all may point to being unable to drive. In terms of 'Class 2' driving, that's driving a bus or lorry, a dementia diagnosis does mean that you need to stop driving this form of vehicle.

It's hard to know if we have been sufficiently impeded by a diagnosis of dementia to stop driving. Fortunately, there are a number of driving assessment centres aimed at those with a disability, physical or mental health diagnosis, that can help take out some of the guesswork when it comes to driving abilities. While the DVLA have the ultimate say on whether we should be driving or not, driving assessment centres can provide a really thorough guide as to whether we still have the skills, awareness, and reactions to operate a motor vehicle.

Now, my wife's car can practically drive itself. You push a few buttons, and it basically follows the car in front, changes speed, keeps to the lanes, and it can even talk. When I was a child, I used to watch a TV programme about a talking car. It seemed like the most amazing thing ever, especially to my young, developing mind. Now my wife's car does it. That said, I don't think the car in the programme was full of quite so many crumbs or toys from the front of magazines as my wife's car is.

You can find more information about driving assessment centres in the Bibliography section at the end of the book.

10
Living with dementia

To some extent, this whole book is about living with dementia. For some, being diagnosed with dementia is like a bolt from the blue. For others, particularly loved ones, it comes as no surprise. The question is, how do we go about life with such a diagnosis? We have seen that dementia isn't about medications. There are some, and they work a bit, but they merely slow down the progression of the condition rather than give us back what's gone. They help reduce the burden of the symptoms, but the end result is the same. When or if a cure for dementia arrives, I'm sure there's a Nobel Prize in the offing.

How do we live with dementia? We just live with dementia. Knowing the diagnosis is really about forearming ourselves, planning for the future. We might have an idea of where that will lead, but it's just an idea. Tomorrow isn't written. Consider a diagnosis as a plot outline, but the detail is yet to be filled in. There's no script.

Living with dementia is living. So get on with it. Do things you enjoy, and don't put them off. Spend time with the people you love. Spend time, don't kill it. I've always wondered why we use the term 'killing time'. Surely it's time that's killing us.

Take all offers of help you can, even if it isn't quite the sort of help you want. Build a world around you that's as future proof as you can make it. Fill the house with aide memoires, and make it safe. Grab rails, raised steps, bathroom adaptations, pendant alarms, easier to use appliances, key safes to permit service providers to come in and help. If you like gardening, get raised beds, flat paths and easy to maintain plants. Whatever hobby you have, keep doing it for as long as you can. Like painting? Who cares what it may look like, just paint. Sing, dance, go for long walks with the people you care about and love. Think about respite for the ones who might look out for you or look after you.

I get to leave my patients at the clinic, but for those of us caring for our loved one, there's little headspace or time to ourselves. This is especially the case as dementia develops.

Think about future mobility. If you might need to give up driving, perhaps consider moving closer to services. I work in a very rural area, and meet a lot of people who 'retire to the countryside'. I like a bit of fresh air and greenery myself, but retiring to the countryside has always seemed like a bad idea to me. The suburbs is where it's at. Leafy green pastures far off the beaten track are of no use if you can't drive. Needing oil delivered is of no use if you're struggling to manage your finances. Living far away from the doctors, dentists, or social activities is of no use if the bus runs twice a day, and you need to walk down a pathless country road to the bus stop. Like I say, move to the suburbs.

Think about social activities. Loneliness is a common problem among older people, and most dementias are more common the older we get. Yet I meet so many people who, to some degree or another, suffer from social isolation. The great thing is there's usually loads of stuff going on in your local area for people in a similar situation.

I used to work in a small, rural market town during the early stages of my career. There was what was nominally called a day centre. For some, the concept of a day centre is like the older person's version of a kindergarten, except with fewer toys and more tea and biscuits. The day centre where I worked was amazing. You could get transport there, there was always something on, it had a fully licensed bar that made student union prices seem expensive, and you could even have a hot bath there, with help from carers if needed. It's still going even to this day. They also have a barbers, a beauty salon, a computer class, a chiropodist, exercise classes, Tai Chi and a hearing aid clinic.

The thing is, these places exist, and you just need to find out more about them. The chances are there's something similar near you.

Dementia is a disease of families. There's something that can be particularly cruel about it, and it can put a lot of strain on loved ones. Dementia, particularly Alzheimer's, isn't always apparent to the person suffering from it. Particularly in the early stages. It's not unusual to see someone in clinic who has no idea why they are there, not because they've forgotten, but because they see their memory as without deficit. It's only when you start asking a few questions that these problems become all too apparent.

11
Making plans (for Nanna) and carers

Dementia care is all about making plans. Hoping for the best, preparing for otherwise. So think about a few things well in advance. Think about power of attorney, as mentioned previously, and think about your living environment. Consider what happens if your loved ones are unavailable, and perhaps consider getting carers in or booking respite. Many residential homes take people for a week or so while their loved ones get a well-earned break. This can usually be arranged directly with the home and, while is isn't always cheap, never underestimate the value of feeling rested, both as a carer and as someone with dementia.

Think about what happens if you need to go into hospital. Hospitals are confusing places. I'm quite happy in them, but I literally lived in a hospital for years. To me, they're one of my happy places. Being admitted to a hospital, at least in the UK, only happens when you absolutely have to go in. We don't admit people to a hospital for the fun of it, particularly as they're incredibly busy and often filled to bursting point.

Having dementia can be confusing and disorientating. Whisk someone off in the middle of the night to a busy, noisy Emergency Department or admissions unit, and it is no wonder we might feel confused. It's worth having a little pack together in case of emergencies. A folder with details about medical problems, emergency contact details such as next of kin, a list of medications and allergies, particularly if you can't quite remember all the details or your loved one or carer is unavailable at the time of admission. Many areas across the UK have packs of this sort of information, and in my patch it's called a 'yellow folder'. Because it's yellow. It contains details of health problems, carer preferences as discussed with the patient, next-of-kin or power of attorney, and a 'do not attempt cardiopulmonary resuscitation'

(DNACPR) form. It helps people know what your preferences are if you're admitted in a hurry.

Think about death. While this might come as a bit of a surprise to some, we're all just temporary. Passing through. Eventually we'll pass away, we will be ex-people, we will cease to be. Planning for the future involves thinking about our ultimate demise. This isn't just about thinking what hymns we might want or whether we want flowers or donations to the cat shelter. It's about where we'd prefer to be cared for in our final weeks or days; what we do and don't want to happen; whether we'd prefer to avoid hospital admissions; whether we want to go to a hospice or stay at home. All of these things should really be thought about in advance, and preferably while we are still in a position to voice these views. Some people might go as far as getting an advanced directive via a solicitor but, as a family doctor in the UK, I don't see these very often.

It's worth having your emergency folder somewhere obvious. I have met people who take them everywhere they go. I've met people who keep theirs in the fridge. As someone who regularly responds to people with urgent medical problems, the fridge isn't always the first place I look in. Keep it somewhere safe and let people know about it.

You might want to consider a medical alert bracelet. These are items of jewelry, such as a necklace or bracelet, often with an inscription outlining allergies or major medical problems. I'd suggest this to anyone with a long-term medical problem or allergy. I'm penicillin allergic. I get an itchy red rash if I have it. I'm pretty sure my wife has forgotten, so maybe I should get one. They're not very expensive and easily obtained.

Being a carer

I really enjoy being a doctor. I am utterly exhausted at the end of every day, there's more work to do than time to do it, and everyone I meet is ill. I mean seriously, it's a wonder anyone is actually alive and in one piece. But as a doctor, by and large, my work stays in the clinic. I might worry about my patients at times outside work, but they aren't sat at the dinner table with me, or coming on holiday at weekends, or phoning me asking me where I am, and can someone walk the dog. Being a family carer is a different matter. The relationship changes, slowly, steadily and inexorably. The relationship changes from husband and wife, or father and daughter, to nurse and patient.

For some, there's a lot of anxiety and guilt tied up with being a family carer. On the one hand, we might feel a great deal of obligation, a need to help our loved one because they are just that, someone we love. A parent, grandparent, partner or sibling. On the other hand, looking after people is exhausting. Constantly giving a bit of yourself to others means there's little left for yourself. As doctors, we are all too aware of burnout. I've burned out myself. You get to a point where you just can't give anymore. Where one more demand on your time is like a 'wafer thin mint'. Death by a thousand cuts. Another 'quick question', another 'can you just nip to the shops', another 'I've forgotten to collect my meds', another 'can you just take me to the toilet?'. Carer stress is a real thing and, over time, being a family carer builds a degree of resentment. Just as it's not my patient's fault they are ill, neither is it our loved one's fault they are needed. But we must be our own patient first. We are not superheroes, even if what we do as carers seems heroic. Carers soak up a lot of needs, a lot of demand, that would otherwise fall to statutory services. They keep people well, fed, hydrated, clean, in their own homes, out of hospital and, often, loved.

Being a carer is difficult. It brings with it a real risk of illness, both physical and mental. I've met people who've neglected their own needs so much that they themselves have become unwell, be it physical or mental. Every cup overflows, and as they say on the plane during the safety announcement, 'put your own mask on before helping others'. It's a good analogy. But that mask shouldn't be one of pretence, of just saying 'I'm okay', when you're not. Depression, anxiety, physical health problems, all are possible as a carer. This doesn't just go for unpaid family carers, but professionals too. We are all vulnerable to illness. We are none of us immune.

So, where's this all leading to? Get help, as much as you can, as often as you can, and don't be afraid to ask for it. People like me aren't going to hunt you down. Social workers aren't going to pop by on the off chance that you might need a bit of help. You've got to 'fess up and admit that help is needed.

The question is, what help is out there? How do we know that we might need care? Sometimes it isn't obvious till it's really obvious, like a trip to the hospital or an accident happening. How do we even get care?

Getting Care

How do we know if we need care? It's a difficult question to answer, particularly if we don't quite have the insight to notice where our memory might be failing. In general terms, I would suggest that if there's something we are struggling to do, we need to get help with it. In terms of physical care, this could be carrying out activities such as gardening or cleaning, going shopping or preparing meals. It might be more fundamental needs such as getting washed or dressed, or going to the toilet. There are several levels of care, and exactly how much we need is often hard to estimate. That said, social services departments are usually the first place I point people in the direction of when it comes to wondering about care.

In my experience, there's a sort of hierarchy of care and, I hasten to add, this is based on my experience, and not really on any particular model or service. As a general rule of thumb, the more care you need, the more it's going to cost.

- No care - everything is fine, nothing to see here.
- Gardener and cleaner - usually privately sourced, you're pretty much OK but just need a bit of help. Or you live at Downton Abbey.
- Carer a couple of times a week - usually to help with bathing, but could be anything you might need help with on a couple of occasions in the week.
- Once daily carer - a short visit, usually with one person, often to help with a particular need. It might be simply to help with lunch, or perhaps medications.

- Twice daily carer - perhaps you need help getting in or out of bed, or someone to help get you breakfast or evening meals.
- Three times a day carer - often helping with meals, medications or personal care.
- Four times a day carer - pretty much the 'top dose' of social care, where someone comes round four times a day to attend to personal needs, often encompassing bedtime routines, ablutions, medications and meals.
- Night carers - someone to come and help overnight. I've seen this used perhaps intermittently for people who have family members who tend to wander at night or become agitated.
- 24 hour care - someone present all around the clock, often working in shifts, but in some cases they move in.

Once you're at the 24 hour care level, your need is usually quite high and, in general, this doesn't come cheap. Social care is usually privately funded, meaning you'll need to pay for it yourself. In the UK, healthcare, the sort of thing I do for people, is free at the point of delivery. This isn't the case in many parts of the world. Social care, personal care and help with everyday activities, is funded by the person using them.

Many carers come via a care agency. It's often difficult to know what agency to go to, particularly if you're researching this yourself. Many may be recommended by the local social services department. Some people I meet go into private arrangements, using a team of regular, private carers to cater to their needs, and this can work well.

After increased home care, the next step is residential care of some form. This might be intermittent and occasional, such as respite care, and it might be permanent. The decision of whether to move into some form of supported living environment is one that isn't taken lightly, and can bring with it considerable anxiety. It's a big wrench for many. Over life we create ties. Ties to people, places, buildings, things, ways of life, hobbies, interests, and even our sense of self. Dementia changes this. People change, you might need to move, you can't take all your stuff with you, your hobbies may change in line with changing abilities, and who you think you actually are is something different. We all change, we are all impermanent, and the things we acquire throughout life are no more or less permanent than we are. I don't mean this to sound depressing, just real. 'You can't take it with you', and the same is said for that chest of drawers you were rather fond of. It's only stuff.

The ties that are the strongest are the hardest to break, and yet we all need to change the things we are tied to. Moving into a residential setting, be it in housing with care, warden controlled, your own place in a senior living complex, or even a nursing home, is a nerve-wracking experience. It's also often rather expensive, so be prepared for that.

Sometimes we have to be really honest with ourselves, and our carers or loved ones, that now's the time to get extra support in the form of residential placement. It's usually better done when we are well, and able to voice our concerns. I see way too many people who end up getting placed somewhere that might not have been their first choice as a result of a hospital admission. Usually a fall, trip and slip, a fracture, an infection, a bit of confusion, a delayed discharge and a 'not quite being as well as you were before' and, before you know it, not quite able to stay at home.

How we go about choosing a home can be quite challenging. You might already have friends, family members or loved ones that live somewhere and like it. You might have recommendations. Like any choice in life, it's worth doing your homework. Probably the best way of getting a feel of how things are is visiting a few places, and spending time talking to the residents. The Care Quality Commission inspects health and social care establishments regularly, and the ratings can be found on their website.

I'm not an expert in residential care. I see a lot, but it's often on home visits to see patients. This always seems to coincide with lunchtime, which isn't the best time to interrupt anyone. Or the night. So it's hard to get a handle on whether a place is good or not. That said, there are a few things I think are worth considering.

Naturally, cost will need to be considered, and many homes and care settings are not cheap. It's not a surprise too, given that they have to combine care with comfort, have staff present 24/7, and regularly renew fixtures and fittings, decor, carpets, etc.

Ask about the staff. Is there a high staff turnover? If staff don't stay long, I would wonder what sort of place it is to work. Remember they're not just homes, but places of work and businesses too and, if something seems a bit fishy, it might be worth digging deeper. If the staff are all long served, not only does it suggest a happy workforce but also good continuity of care. Have a wander around, talk to the staff, other residents, and other family members. The best way of getting an idea about how good a place to live in is, is to ask those that already do.

Summary

I hope that, despite the challenges you've faced, are facing, and are yet to face, that this book has been useful. Any diagnosis can be scary, but it's just that. A diagnosis. It doesn't define you, but it might just change the future to one that was perhaps a little less planned. Knowing a bit about dementia, causes, treatments and how to get help can hopefully shed a little light on what can otherwise be scary. Fear comes from the unknown, the 'what if', the unsaid. Hopefully I've been able to shed a little light into the darker recesses of that fear.

I don't think I've met anyone who has been untouched by dementia. We've had several family members develop it. Vascular, mixed, and I'm pretty sure Lewy body is in there too. Like I say, we are none of us immune.

Experiences of dementia vary widely. I've looked after a lot of people with dementia at varying stages. Some I've met crack on with life, keep on doing what they enjoy, and adapt to the disease. Some I've met spend their entire time laughing and joking. One chap I meet on a regular basis is somewhat flirty, with pretty much everyone, but once again is laughing and joking. One lady I met repeatedly was in constant good spirits but did leave me thinking I might need a chaperone for my own safety. She was in her eighties. I'm still not sure how to view her advances. She once randomly stroked me on the back as she left the room. I've also had people fail to recognize their loved ones, their house, or realize where they are and make a dash for it, much to the distress of those around.

If there's a take home message I can provide it's this: get help. Take all the help you can when it's offered, and if it isn't offered then seek it out. Regardless of the condition, be it dementia, cancer, a broken bone or man-flu, we can all get by with a little help from our friends. And occupational therapy. And meals on wheels. And the chiropodist. And social services. You get the picture.

What does the future hold for dementia? Organizations such as Alzheimer's Research UK are helping fund studies across the world in order to discover more about the causes and treatment of dementia, as well as how we might be able to prevent it from happening in the first place. In time, we will understand more about the many causes of dementia, be able to recognize it in advance and, hopefully, stop the condition from progressing before it becomes a problem.

Being diagnosed with dementia can be a really scary proposition, but it doesn't have to be. There is a lot of help out there, and you just need to know where to look. Hopefully this book has helped provide a little more insight into the condition, and help show you how to get that help, when needed.

Useful Resources

Living with dementia isn't easy, but you are not alone. The following are useful links to organizations that can be of help. They're correct at the time of writing, but with many organizations and links, time can lead them to change. This list is no means exhaustive but might provide a useful starting point. Feel free to scribble extra useful links in the margins. That's what they're for.

1   Your local social services department. They're a very useful source of help, especially when it comes to getting help and support in terms of care.

2   Your local doctor's surgery. It sounds like a cliché but it is true. Book an appointment.

3   Dementia UK. A charity providing specialized nurses, among other services.
    Dementia UK Head Office
    7th Floor
    One Aldgate
    London EC3N 1RE
    Tel.: 0800 888 6678
    Website: www.dementiauk.org

4   Alzheimer's Society. National charity covering many types of dementia.
    43–44 Crutched Friars
    London EC3N 2AE
    Tel.: 0300 222 1122
    Website: www.alzheimers.org.uk

5   Age UK. National charity covering all areas of life affecting older people.
    Tavis House
    1–6 Tavistock Square
    London WC1H 9NA
    Tel.: 0800 678 1602
    Website: www.ageuk.org.uk

6   The Lewy Body Society. UK based charity covering DLB.
    The Lewy Body Society
    Unity House
    Westwood Park
    Wigan WN3 4HE
    Tel.: 0800 888 6678
    Website: www.lewybody.org

7   Alzheimer's Association. US based charity.
    225 N. Michigan Ave.
    Floor 17
    Chicago, IL 60601 USA
    Tel.: 800 .272 .3900
    Website: www.alz.org

8   Mental Health Foundation. UK based charity for all areas of
    mental illness.
    Colechurch House
    1 London Bridge Walk
    London SE1 2SX
    Tel.: 020 7803 1100
    Website: www.mentalhealth.org.uk

9   Alzheimer's Research UK. UK based research charity.
    Alzheimer's Research UK
    3 Riverside
    Granta Park
    Cambridge. CB21 6AD
    Tel.: 0300 111 5555
    Website: www.alzheimersresearchuk.org

10 Parkinson's UK. UK based PD charity.
    215 Vauxhall Bridge Road
    London. SW1V 1EJ
    Tel.: 0808 800 0303
    Website: www.parkinsons.org.uk

Bibliography

Alzheimer's Research UK. About MCI.
www.alzheimersresearchuk.org/about-dementia/types-of-dementia/mild-cognitive-impairment/about/

Alzheimer Society Calgary. About Alzheimer's & Dementia.
www.alzheimercalgary.ca/about-alzheimers-and-dementia/types-of-dementia/mixed-dementia

Abraha, I., Rimland, J. M., Lozano-Montoya, I., Dell'aquila, G., Vélez-Díaz-Pallarés, M., Trotta, F. M., Cruz-Jentoft, A. J., Cherubini, A., 2017. *Simulated presence therapy for dementia*. Cochrane Database of Systematic Reviews.
doi:10.1002/14651858.cd011882.pub2

Advances in Our Understanding of the Pathophysiology of Alzheimer's Disease, 2011. touchNEUROLOGY.
www.touchneurology.com/articles/advances-our-understanding-pathophysiology-alzheimers-disease

Alzheimer's Disease Fact Sheet. National Institute on Aging.
www.nia.nih.gov/health/alzheimers-disease-fact-sheet

Alzheimer's Disease Genetics Fact Sheet. National Institute on Aging.
www.nia.nih.gov/health/alzheimers-disease-genetics-fact-sheet

Alzheimer's Society's view on demography. Alzheimer's Society.
www.alzheimers.org.uk/info/20091/what_we_think/93/demography

Alzheimer's disease, 2018. Mayo Clinic.
www.mayoclinic.org/diseases-conditions/alzheimers-disease/symptoms-causes/syc-20350447

Alzheimer's disease: Overview, 2017. InformedHealth.org.
www.ncbi.nlm.nih.gov/books/NBK279360/

Antipsychotic drugs. Alzheimer's Society.
www.alzheimers.org.uk/about-dementia/treatments/drugs/antipsychotic-drugs

Aricept Tablets - Summary of Product Characteristics (SmPC). EMC.
www.medicines.org.uk/emc/product/3776/smpc

Baillon, S. F., Narayana, U., Luxenberg, J. S., Clifton, A. V., 2018. *Valproate preparations for agitation in dementia*. Cochrane Database of Systematic Reviews.
doi:10.1002/14651858.cd003945.pub4

Barkhof, F., van Buchem, M. A., 2016. *Neuroimaging in Dementia*. Diseases of the Brain, Head and Neck, Spine. p79–85. doi:10.1007/978-3-319-30081-8_10

Brain Structure and Function: TBI Basics. braininjuryeducation.org/TBI-Basics/Brain-Structure-and-Function/

BrainMade Simple. Hippocampus. brainmadesimple.com/hippocampus.html

Bryant, J., Clegg, A., Nicholson, T., Mcintyre, L., Broe, S. D., Gerard, K., Waugh, N., 2001. *Clinical and cost-effectiveness of donepezil, rivastigmine and galantamine for Alzheimer's disease: a rapid and systematic review*. Health Technology Assessment 5. doi:10.3310/hta5010

Buschert, V., Bokde, A. L. W., Hampel, H., 2010. *Cognitive intervention in Alzheimer disease*. Nature News. www.nature.com/articles/nrneurol.2010.113

Causes and Risk Factors of Alzheimer's Disease. WebMD. www.webmd.com/alzheimers/guide/alzheimers-causes-risk-factors

Computed Tomography (CT). National Institute of Biomedical Imaging and Bioengineering. www.nibib.nih.gov/science-education/science-topics/computed-tomography-ct

Corticobasal Degeneration. NORD (National Organization for Rare Disorders). rarediseases.org/rare-diseases/corticobasal-degeneration/

D'onofrio, G., Sancarlo, D., Seripa, D., Ricciardi, F., Giuliani, F., Panza, F., Greco, A., 2016. *Non-Pharmacological Approaches in the Treatment of Dementia*. Update on Dementia. doi:10.5772/64232

Dam, P. H. V., Caljouw, M. A., Slettebø, D. D., Achterberg, W. P., Husebo, B. S., *Quality of Life and Pain Medication Use in Persons With Advanced Dementia Living in Long-Term Care Facilities*. Journal of the American Medical Directors Association. doi:10.1016/j.jamda.2019.02.019

Dementia. World Health Organization. www.who.int/en/news-room/fact-sheets/detail/dementia

Dementia UK report. Alzheimer's Society. www.alzheimers.org.uk/info/20025/policy_and_influencing/251/dementia_uk

Dementia with Lewy Bodies. DLB information. Patient.info. patient.info/doctor/dementia-with-lewy-bodies

Donaghy, P. C., Mckeith, I. G., 2014. *The clinical characteristics of dementia with Lewy bodies and a consideration of prodromal diagnosis*. Alzheimer's Research & Therapy 6, p46. doi:10.1186/alzrt274

Douglas, S., James, I., Ballard, C., 2004. *Non-pharmacological interventions in dementia*. Advances in Psychiatric Treatment 10, p171–177. doi:10.1192/apt.10.3.171

Driving with dementia or mild cognitive impairment: Consensus guidelines for clinicians. British Geriatrics Society, 2019. www.bgs.org.uk/resources/driving-with-dementia-or-mild-cognitive-impairment-consensus-guidelines-for-clinicians

Dyer, S. M., Harrison, S. L., Laver, K., Whitehead, C., Crotty, M. *An overview of systematic reviews of pharmacological and non-pharmacological interventions for the treatment of behavioral and psychological symptoms of dementia*. International Psychogeriatrics 30, p295–309. doi:10.1017/s1041610217002344

Farina, N., Llewellyn, D., Mokhtar Gad El Kareem Nasr Isaac, Tabet, N., 2017. *Vitamin E for Alzheimer's dementia and mild cognitive impairment*. Cochrane Database of Systematic Reviews. doi:10.1002/14651858.cd002854.pub5

Flicker, L., Evans, J. G., 2004. *Piracetam for dementia or cognitive impairment*. Cochrane Database of Systematic Reviews. doi:10.1002/14651858.cd001011

Flier, W. M. V. D., Skoog, I., Schneider, J. A., Pantoni, L., Mok, V., Chen, C. L. H., Scheltens, P., 2018. *Vascular cognitive impairment*. Nature Reviews Disease Primers 4. doi:10.1038/nrdp.2018.3

Forrester, L. T., Maayan, N., Orrell, M., Spector, A. E., Buchan, L. D., Soares-Weiser, K., 2014. *Aromatherapy for dementia*. Cochrane Database of Systematic Reviews. doi:10.1002/14651858.cd003150.pub2

Frontotemporal dementia. Alzheimer's Disease and Dementia. www.alz.org/alzheimers-dementia/what-is-dementia/types-of-dementia/frontotemporal-dementia

Frontotemporal dementia. Rare Dementia Support. www.raredementiasupport.org/ftd/

Frontotemporal dementia: what is it? Alzheimer's Society. www.alzheimers.org.uk/about-dementia/types-dementia/frontotemporal-dementia

Garcia-Esparcia, P., López-González, I., Grau-Rivera, O., García-Garrido, M. F., Konetti, A., Llorens, F., Zafar, S., Carmona, M., Rio, J. A. D., Zerr, I., Gelpi, E., Ferrer, I., 2017. *Dementia with Lewy Bodies: Molecular Pathology in the Frontal Cortex in Typical and Rapidly Progressive Forms.* Frontiers in Neurology 8. doi:10.3389/fneur.2017.00089

Getting involved in research. Alzheimer's Research UK. www.alzheimersresearchuk.org/about-dementia/helpful-information/getting-involved-in-research/

Home. Alzheimer's Disease and Dementia. www.alz.org/

Home: Lewy Body Dementia Association. www.lbda.org/

Hoz, L. D., Simons, M., 2014. *The emerging functions of oligodendrocytes in regulating neuronal network behaviour.* BioEssays 37, p60–69. doi:10.1002/bies.201400127

Huntington's Disease. Huntington's Disease Association. www.hda.org.uk/professionals/about-huntingtons

Introduction to posterior cortical atrophy. Rare Dementia Support. www.raredementiasupport.org/pca/what-is-pca/intro-to-pca/

Jabr, F., 2012. Know Your Neurons: How to Classify Different Types of Neurons in the Brain's Forest . Scientific American Blog Network. blogs.scientificamerican.com/brainwaves/know-your-neurons-classifying-the-many-types-of-cells-in-the-neuron-forest/

Janelidze, M., Botchorishvili, N., 2018. *Mild Cognitive Impairment.* Alzheimer's Disease - The 21st Century Challenge. doi:10.5772/intechopen.75509

Key Findings. Cognitive Function and Ageing Studies. www.cfas.ac.uk/cfas-i/cfasi-key-findings/

Kirchner, V., Kelly, C. A., Harvey, R. J., 2001. *Thioridazine for dementia.* Cochrane Database of Systematic Reviews. doi:10.1002/14651858.cd000464

Krishnan, S., Cairns, R., Howard, R., 2009. *Cannabinoids for the treatment of dementia.* Cochrane Database of Systematic Reviews. doi:10.1002/14651858.cd007204.pub2

Learn Genetics. The Other Brain Cells. learngendev.azurewebsites.net/content/neuroscience/braincells/

Lewy Body Dementia. Patient.info.
   patient.info/health/memory-loss-and-dementia/lewy-body-
   dementia
Lewy Body Dementia. MedlinePlus.
   medlineplus.gov/lewybody-disease.html
Magnetic Resonance Imaging (MRI). National Institute of
   Biomedical Imaging and Bioengineering.
   www.nibib.nih.gov/science-education/science-topics/magnetic-
   resonance-imaging-mri
Masters, C. L., Bateman, R., Blennow, K., Rowe, C. C., Sperling,
   R. A., Cummings, J. L., 2015. *Alzheimer's disease*. Nature News.
   www.nature.com/articles/nrdp201556
Mawanda, F., Wallace, R., 2013. *Can Infections Cause Alzheimer's
   Disease?* OUP Academic.
   academic.oup.com/epirev/article/35/1/161/551808
Mccleery, J., Cohen, D. A., Sharpley, A. L., 2016. *Pharmacotherapies
   for sleep disturbances in dementia*. Cochrane Database of
   Systematic Reviews.
   doi:10.1002/14651858.cd009178.pub3
Mcguinness, B., Cardwell, C. R., Passmore, P., 2016. *Statin
   withdrawal in people with dementia*. Cochrane Database of
   Systematic Reviews.
   doi:10.1002/14651858.cd012050.pub2
Memory and thinking. Multiple Sclerosis Society UK.
   www.mssociety.org.uk/about-ms/signs-and-symptoms/
   memory-and-thinking
Memory, Learning, and Emotion: the Hippocampus. PsychEducation.
   psycheducation.org/brain-tours/memory-learning-and-
   emotion-the-hippocampus/
Mild Cognitive Impairment. Memory and Aging Center.
   memory.ucsf.edu/mild-cognitive-impairment
Mild Cognitive Impairment. MedlinePlus.
   medlineplus.gov/mildcognitiveimpairment.html
Mild Cognitive Impairment. Alzheimer's Society.
   www.alzheimers.org.uk/about-dementia/types-dementia/mild-
   cognitive-impairment-mci
Mixed Dementia. Dementia.org.
   www.dementia.org/mixed-dementia
Mixed Dementia. Alzheimer's Association.
   www.alz.org/alzheimers-dementia/what-is-dementia/types-of-
   dementia/mixed-dementia

Mortimer, A. M., Likeman, M., Lewis, T. T., 2013. *Neuroimaging in dementia: a practical guide.* Practical Neurology 13, p92–103. doi:10.1136/practneurol-2012-000337

Murphy, E., Froggatt, K., Connolly, S., O'shea, E., Sampson, E. L., Casey, D., Devane, D., 2016. *Palliative care interventions in advanced dementia.* Cochrane Database of Systematic Reviews. doi:10.1002/14651858.cd011513.pub2

Nelson, D., 2019. *Cerebrum: Function Of The Largest Part Of The Human Brain.* Science Trends. sciencetrends.com/cerebrum-functions-largest-part-human-brain/

Neuroimaging in dementia: an update for the general clinician Progress in Neurology and Psychiatry. www.progressnp.com/article/neuroimaging-dementia-update-general-clinician/

Neuroscience Online: An Electronic Textbook for the Neurosciences. Department of Neurobiology and Anatomy - The University of Texas Medical School at Houston. nba.uth.tmc.edu/neuroscience/index.htm

New avenues for brain repair poster. Abcam. www.abcam.com/neuroscience/new-avenues-for-brain-repair-poster

Non-drug approaches to certain symptoms. Alzheimer's Society. www.alzheimers.org.uk/about-dementia/treatments/drugs/non-drug-approaches

Non-drug interventions for Alzheimer's disease. InformedHealth. org. www.ncbi.nlm.nih.gov/books/NBK279355/#_PMH0072539_pubdet_

Olazarán, J., Reisberg, B., Clare, L., Cruz, I., Peña-Casanova, J., Ser, T. D., Woods, B., Beck, C., Auer, S., Lai, C., Spector, A., Fazio, S., Bond, J., Kivipelto, M., Brodaty, H., Rojo, J. M., Collins, H., Teri, L., Mittelman, M., Orrell, M., Feldman, H. H., Muñiz, R., 2010. *Nonpharmacological Therapies in Alzheimer's Disease: A Systematic Review of Efficacy.* Dementia and Geriatric Cognitive Disorders 30, p161–178. doi:10.1159/000316119

Oliveira, A. M. D., Radanovic, M., Mello, P. C. H. D., Buchain, P. C., Vizzotto, A. D. B., Celestino, D. L., Stella, F., Piersol, C. V., Forlenza, O. V., 2015. *Nonpharmacological Interventions to Reduce Behavioral and Psychological Symptoms of Dementia: A Systematic Review.* BioMed Research International 2015, p1–9. doi:10.1155/2015/218980

Overview: Donepezil, galantamine, rivastigmine and memantine for the treatment of Alzheimer's disease: Guidance. NICE. www.nice.org.uk/guidance/ta217

Parkinson's Disease Dementia. Memory and Aging Center. memory.ucsf.edu/dementia/parkinsons/parkinson-disease-dementia

Petersen, R. C., Lopez, O., Armstrong, M. J., Getchius, T. S., Ganguli, M., Gloss, D., Gronseth, G. S., Marson, D., Pringsheim, T., Day, G. S., Sager, M., Stevens, J., Rae-Grant, A., 2017. *Practice guideline update summary: Mild cognitive impairment.* Neurology 90, p126–135.
doi:10.1212/wnl.0000000000004826

Poewe, W., Gauthier, S., Aarsland, D., Leverenz, J. B., Barone, P., Weintraub, D., Tolosa, E., Dubois, B., 2008. *Diagnosis and management of Parkinson's disease dementia.* International Journal of Clinical Practice 62, p1581–1587.
doi:10.1111/j.1742-1241.2008.01869.x

Possible Causes of Alzheimer's Disease. BrightFocus Foundation. www.brightfocus.org/alzheimers/article/possible-causes-alzheimers-disease

Posterior Cortical Atrop [. Alzheimer's Disease and Dementia. www.alz.org/alzheimers-dementia/what-is-dementia/types-of-dementia/posterior-cortical-atrophy

Prescribing drugs for Alzheimer's disease in primary care: managing cognitive symptoms: Table, 2014. Drug and Therapeutics Bulletin 52, p69–72.
doi:10.1136/dtb.2014.6.0261

Prevalence. Dementia Statistics Hub. www.dementiastatistics.org/statistics-about-dementia/prevalence/

Price, J. D., Hermans, D., Evans, J. G., 2001. *Subjective barriers to prevent wandering of cognitively impaired people.* Cochrane Database of Systematic Reviews.
doi:10.1002/14651858.cd001932

Primary Progressive Aphasia. Memory and Aging Center. memory.ucsf.edu/dementia/primary-progressive-aphasia

Primary Progressive Aphasia or PPA. AFTD. www.theaftd.org/what-is-ftd/primary-progressive-aphasia/

Primary progressive aphasia. Genetic and Rare Diseases Information Center. rarediseases.info.nih.gov/diseases/8541/primary-progressive-aphasia

Przedborski, S., Vila, M., Jackson-Lewis, V., 2003. *Series Introduction: Neurodegeneration: What is it and where are we?* Journal of Clinical Investigation 111, p3–10.
doi:10.1172/jci200317522

Psychiatry CPD. Neuroimaging in dementia.
www.psychiatrycpd.co.uk/learningmodules/neuroimagingin-dementia.aspx

Publications. Cognitive Function and Ageing Studies.
www.cfas.ac.uk/publications/

Recommendations: Dementia: assessment, management and support for people living with dementia and their carers: Guidance. NICE.
www.nice.org.uk/guidance/ng97/chapter/Recommendations#interventions-to-promote-cognition-independence-and-wellbeing

Research - Clinical Trials Watch. Alzheimer Europe.
www.alzheimer-europe.org/Research/Clinical-Trials-Watch

Roberts, M., 2018. *Alzheimer's researchers win brain prize.* BBC News.
www.bbc.co.uk/news/health-43300185

Rostad, H. M., Utne, I., Grov, E. K., Småstuen, M. C., Puts, M., Halvorsrud, L., 2018. *The impact of a pain assessment intervention on pain score and analgesic use in older nursing home residents with severe dementia: A cluster randomised controlled trial.* International Journal of Nursing Studies 84, p52–60.
doi:10.1016/j.ijnurstu.2018.04.017

Royal Society for Public Health UK.
www.rsph.org.uk/

Sajjadi, S. A., Brown, J., Clinical assessment of patients with dementia. ACNR Online Neurology Journal RSS2.
www.acnr.co.uk/2015/09/clinical-assessment-of-patients-with-dementia/

Search Statistics. Dementia Statistics Hub.
www.dementiastatistics.org/search-statistics/

Search of: Alzheimer Disease - List Results. ClinicalTrials.gov.
www.clinicaltrials.gov/ct2/results?cond=Alzheimer+Disease&term=&cntry=&state=&city=&dist=

Squire, L. R., Horst, A. S. V. D., Mcduff, S. G. R., Frascino, J. C., Hopkins, R. O., Mauldin, K. N., 2010. *Role of the hippocampus in remembering the past and imagining the future.* Proceedings of the National Academy of Sciences 107.
doi:10.1073/pnas.1014391107

Stinton, C., Mckeith, I., Taylor, J.-P., Lafortune, L., Mioshi, E., Mak, E., Cambridge, V., Mason, J., Thomas, A., O'Brien, J. T., 2015.

Pharmacological Management of Lewy Body Dementia: A Systematic Review and Meta-Analysis. American Journal of Psychiatry 172, p731–742.
doi:10.1176/appi.ajp.2015.14121582

Szatmári, S., Bereczki, D., 2008. *Procaine treatments for cognition and dementia.* Cochrane Database of Systematic Reviews.
doi:10.1002/14651858.cd005993.pub2

Take part in research studies. Alzheimer's Society.
www.alzheimers.org.uk/research/play-your-part/participate-in-research

Takeda, M., Tanaka, T., Okochi, M., Kazui, H., 2012. *Non-pharmacological intervention for dementia patients.* Psychiatry and Clinical Neurosciences 66, p1–7.
doi:10.1111/j.1440-1819.2011.02304.x

Tips for dealing with memory and thinking problems. Multiple Sclerosis Society UK.
www.mssociety.org.uk/about-ms/signs-and-symptoms/memory-and-thinking/tips-for-dealing-with-memory-and-thinking-problems

UCL - London's Global University. Dementia Research Centre.
www.ucl.ac.uk/drc/current-trials

Wang, H.-F., Yu, J.-T., Tang, S.-W., Jiang, T., Tan, C.-C., Meng, X.-F., Wang, C., Tan, M.-S., Tan, L., 2014. *Efficacy and safety of cholinesterase inhibitors and memantine in cognitive impairment in Parkinson's disease, Parkinson's disease dementia, and dementia with Lewy bodies: systematic review with meta-analysis and trial sequential analysis.* Journal of Neurology, Neurosurgery & Psychiatry 86, p135–143.
doi:10.1136/jnnp-2014-307659

Warren, J. D., Rohrer, J. D., Rossor, M. N., 2013. *Frontotemporal dementia.* BMJ 347.
doi:10.1136/bmj.f4827

Westervelt, H. J., 2015. *Dementia in Multiple Sclerosis: Why Is It Rarely Discussed?* Archives of Clinical Neuropsychology 30, p174–177.
doi:10.1093/arclin/acu095

What Causes Alzheimer's Disease? National Institute on Aging.
www.nia.nih.gov/health/what-causes-alzheimers-disease

Wild, R., Pettit, T. A., Burns, A., 2003. *Cholinesterase inhibitors for dementia with Lewy bodies.* Cochrane Database of Systematic Reviews.
doi:10.1002/14651858.cd003672

Woods, S. P., Moore, D. J., Weber, E., Grant, I., 2009. *Cognitive Neuropsychology of HIV-Associated Neurocognitive Disorders.* Neuropsychology Review 19, p152–168.
doi:10.1007/s11065-009-9102-5

Zupancic, M., Mahajan, A., Handa, K., 2011. Dementia With Lewy Bodies. *The Primary Care Companion For CNS Disorders.* PubMed.
doi:10.4088/pcc.11r01190

The functions of glia in the CNS. Abcam.
www.abcam.com/neuroscience/the-functions-of-glia-in-the-cns

Index